Copyright © 2022 Jerome Vergamini

All rights reserved. No part of this book may be reproduced or transmitted in any form or by any means electronic or mechanical including photocopying, recording, or by any information storage and retrieval system without permission in writing from the publisher.

Aurora Books, an imprint of Eco-Justice Press, L.L.C.

Aurora Books
P.O. Box 5409 Eugene, OR 97405
www.ecojusticepress.com

Quimby's Quandary: A Psychiatrist's Journey
By Jerome Vergamini

Library of Congress Control Number: 2021953537
ISBN 978-1-945432-50-7

Quimby's Quandary
A Psychiatrist's Journey

Jerome Vergamini

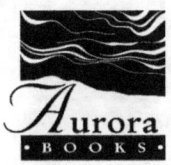

Prologue:
OLD MAN IN THE DOG PARK
March 2021

He unhooked the leash and stopped near the gate to get some poop bags. The big golden retriever wandered in the grass sniffing where the other dogs had left their marks, settled on an area, and did his thing. Fred walked over and picked it up, grateful that he did not have to walk far to retrieve the small pile. He put the bag in the garbage pail conveniently located near the entrance. That task finished, he walked on the path that circled the park to a table with benches under a shade tree. He sat down while the Sam, the dog, continued what Fred called his Facebook routine, sniffing about to find out which dogs and humans had been here. The path had been freshly graveled, which Fred found uncomfortable for walking, so he tended to sit near the path. By doing so, he could have brief conversations with passersby, and Sam could mingle with other dogs and greet their owners with a dog smile, lean against them and hope for some petting, or maybe even a treat. Fred found it interesting that many people had learned his dog's name but did not know his. It was that kind of a place. People were mainly there for the dogs, but over time were increasingly conversant in a chit-chatty way with other owners.

Fred had found over the years that he had something that drew people to him. He had thought about it and surmised that it had to do with his being somewhat quiet and willing to listen, and that he smiled easily. That had been quite helpful to him in his career as a psychiatrist. He had been retired now for about four years. He came to the dog park to get out, get a bit of exercise and give the dog what he needed, but at the same time to be just an older gentleman with his dog, not an expert on human interaction. Yet, at times, his manner seemed to draw that human interaction.

It amazed Fred that among the numerous people who came to the dog park, many were young women. He would joke with friends sometimes that, had he paid attention as a young man about the number of young women who fawned over dogs, he would have made sure to get a puppy. Now he was simply an old man, occasionally giving advice, but only if it was asked for. As a shrink, he learned quickly that even people who asked for advice did not necessarily want it, but, since that is what they were paying him for, he would feel obligated to provide it, and he did.

On this particular day, a young lady, a college student at the local university, was enticed by Sam to pet him. She was intrigued by his 'doggy smile' as he approached to lean against her to be petted. His lips were pressed back, occasionally making some people think he was growling, but his bushy tail was wagging the whole time like a tree limb in a windstorm. She and Fred chatted for a bit. When he learned that she was a student, he mentioned that he had previously worked at the university. When she found that he had worked as a psychiatrist there, she began to get into more personal things.

"I recently broke up with a guy I've been dating. I couldn't trust him. I let him have it good. He apologized, but I had heard it before. The trouble is, I keep thinking about him. He is good looking, he is smart, and he is likely to have a good career, but he lies. He even got himself kicked out of a study group with classmates."

"Well, that says something. It sounds like his colleagues might also have an opinion of him that is similar to yours."

"I think he just wants me to be somehow attached to him, what he wants, regardless of what I might want."

"From my experience, reasonable men tend to want a woman who is independent, thinks for herself, and can be dealt with as a partner, on an equal status. Otherwise, it is like having an anchor instead of a partner."

"Well, that's not him. That's for sure."

"The difficult part of a romantic breakup is separating thinking from feelings. Our head tells us one thing; our heart says something else."

"Yeah, but how do I do that? It's been almost two months. I know I cannot trust him and do not want to reconnect with him, but I feel guilty for treating him so badly."

"Life is full of thorny patches. The way we get through them is to weigh our options, follow the most reasonable solutions we can muster, then move on without looking back, and learn from our mistakes."

She sat quietly for a while, petting Sam. Fred could see her eyes starting to water. Fred spoke up.

"Sometimes when people are hanging on to things, there is a part of it that they do want. That might be the part that they imagined was there, but it turned out not to be. Losing something that felt so real at the time is hard. You like to keep thinking that maybe it was a mistake, because you wanted it to be real."

"I wish there were something I could do to help me to let it go. I guess it was like a mirage. It looked real and I wanted it, but it really wasn't real."

Sometimes people use rituals to let go, like a funeral. It is hard to let go of something you love. Sometimes a ritual allows you to remember that it is gone."

"Maybe I should bury the earrings he got me."

"Well, if they are worth something, maybe you would be tempted to dig them up again. Or you could pawn them and use the money to do something special for a friend. Then if he really wants them back, he can go to the pawn shop and pay for them again."

She laughed at the thought.

Fred smiles. "See, even talking about it has lightened your mood. Whatever you do, be who you are and don't kick yourself about your choices, just learn from them. Be kind to yourself and I think you will sleep better."

"Thanks. Sounds like good advice."

She got up from sitting on the grass and said, "Well, I had better continue my walk, but thank you for listening."

"Just remember, there are people out there who might not be as debonaire, but who are steady and loyal, and will make solid partners."

As she continued around the park perimeter, Fred watched her look back over her shoulder and wave. He then headed back to the front gate. Sam obediently followed. Fred doubted that he would see her again. He hoped the conversation had helped her. He was glad that he did not go into too much detail with her. He suspected that her loss had more to do with being intimate with him, maybe her first time. Opening that envelope for her would bring up more emotion, and that would need more follow up time with her. He knew that was not possible, and he did not want to stir that pot for her. Hopefully, he had planted seeds that she could nurture.

Chapter one:
FIRST DAY
July 1969

Twenty-seven-year-old Fred Quimby had officially been a psychiatrist for an hour. He had just completed the orientation process and was about to enter ward 2E on his initial rotation as a first-year resident in training. He was assigned to a ward at the state hospital across town from the main university campus. He held the keys in his hand, a symbol of power, but he felt far from powerful. In fact, he was quite nervous.

He had experienced one rotation in psychiatry in medical school and had liked it, but he had never been fully in charge of taking care of patients by himself; he had always worked with the resident in command and followed orders. As he turned the key and let himself in, the door automatically locked behind him with a loud click. He pocketed his keys and sauntered up the tiled hallway toward the nursing station when a somewhat grizzled older man approached him as if to ask a question.

"Are you the new doc? Are you going to give me electroshock treatments?"

Not yet knowing what his new duties would be, Quimby fumbled with an answer.

"I really don't know whether I will be doing that or not."

The old guy quickly got agitated and yelled,

"He's here to give me shock treatments! I don't want you to give me shock treatments!"

The next thing Quimby knew, he was ducking a roundhouse right hook as several orderlies came running down the hall to subdue the man known to the staff as Bobbie the Bomber. Bobbie was an ex-boxer who had taken one too many shots to the head in the ring. Things calmed down rather quickly after Bobbie had been given a sedative, but this was Fred Quimby's introduction to 2E. When he arrived safely at the nursing station 20 feet away, he tried to appear unflustered as he met the several orderlies, the head nurse, and a younger, very attractive redhead nurse. Sadie, the older head nurse, introduced him to the others, Ralph, Joe, and Wanda. Wanda, the redhead, showed him around the unit and tried to put him at ease.

"Bobbie gets excited with new faces and change, but by tomorrow he will have forgotten all about his encounter with you. Hopefully, you'll be more at ease by then as well." Wanda walked Fred to a locked door on the unit.

"This will be your office. Make yourself at home. I'll see you in about an hour after you get settled in. Then I'll introduce you to the ward service chief, Dr. Nolan."

Fred unlocked the door to his new digs. It was a 10x10 room with a metal desk, a metal reclining chair on wheels, a phone, a Dictaphone, a small bookcase, a chair for a patient, and an examining table. There were no pictures on the walls. With a mixture of pride and perhaps a little disappointment, he sat in the chair, put his feet on the desk, and found himself clattering onto the floor as he leaned too far back into the chair. It was quite a racket! Quite embarrassed, he quickly got up, sat himself upright in the chair at the desk as though nothing had happened. He was sure that some staff person would be bolting in to see what all the noise was about and that he was OK. To his relief, but also to his surprise, and perhaps to his chagrin, nobody came in. He wondered, if he got in trouble in this office with a patient, who would know?

There was not much to do other than deciding where he might hang a couple of pictures, checking to see if there was a PDR handy, and wondering whether to bring in some of his own books. He checked the drawers, finding them empty except for a few old, discarded pens and pencils, a phone book, and a few leftover small tablets left by pharmaceutical reps. He checked to see if the windows would open. They would not. He left the room; the door locked automatically when closed.

It had only been about half an hour since Wanda had led him to his office. Fred found her again in the nursing station.

"You're back early. Your appointment with Dr. Nolan isn't for another thirty minutes. Why don't I show you around the unit a bit before you meet with him."

They walked into the dayroom, a large lounging area where patients were free to congregate when not engaged in various treatments. There was a couch, several comfortable looking chairs, several small tables with benches, and large windows that, like in his office, would not open. They overlooked the hospital grounds. Wanda pointed out a few of the "notables" among the patients. "The big man in the chair is Mr. Fields. His family was big in the tobacco business, so they named him Chester. He would have been quite a catch for some young lady at one time, but he was involved in a motorcycle accident and has never been quite right since.

The tall man with the beard is Wilfred Donne. He was an English professor whose wife ran off with a plumber, and he never quite got over it. He became quite delusional and saw himself as the embodiment of the poetic spirit. He cannot make up his mind whether his favorite poet is Wilfred Owen or John Donne, but he becomes the persona of various poets, depending on the day and his fancy. He spends a lot of time quoting poetry.

Over there is Little Rudy. He is quite cagey and needs a close watch. He is chronically depressed and periodically tries to kill himself in ineffective, but sometimes ingenious ways.

That fellow over there is John Jacob Farnsworth. He comes from a wealthy family but has been in a lot of legal trouble, and I think he was sent here to be able to plead insanity to some hefty crimes. I especially suspect this because he is excessively fearful of being around all these 'crazy people'. There are more, but you'll get a chance to meet them another time. It's time to meet Dr. Nolan."

Chapter two:
THE CHIEF

As Wanda walked Fred down the hall to Dr. Anthony Nolan's office, he took in the activity on the unit. Some patients wandered about. They passed the man called by everyone "the poet". He looked at Fred and said, "Beware the Jabberwock my son, the jaws that bite, the claws that catch. Beware the Jubjub bird, and shun the frumious Bandersnatch." And then he walked on.

"What was that all about?" he asked Wanda.

She shrugged and said, "I think Mr. Donne is doing his Lewis Carroll imitation."

Wanda knocked on the door, and they entered after hearing, "Come in."

"Dr. Nolan, this is the new resident, Dr. Fred Quimby. You wanted to meet him once he got settled, so I'll leave the two of you alone to get acquainted." She then left, closing the door behind her. Dr. Nolan looked Quimby up and down for a few moments before speaking. The initial silence was a bit unsettling.

"Dr. Quimby, an unusual name. Pray what is the origin? What nationality is such a name as Quimby?"

Fred wanted to ask a similar question of Dr. Nolan, since he was about 6' 2" in height, muscular, had a very dusky skin tone and at about fifty years of age, had a well-manicured salt & pepper beard. However, he wisely just answered the question.

"Actually, the name comes from an Italian word for a kind of red color – vermilion or cinnabar. The word is 'cinabro', but as with many Italian names, it was altered by the officials at Ellis Island who found it easier to say Quimby." My grandfather was from northern Italy, where it is said that there are many redheads resulting from raids by the Vikings led by Frederik Barbarossa, the name given him because of his red beard."

"All right, all right, I wasn't looking for an exposition from the Encyclopedia Britannica. Let me tell you about your duties here and the expectations. We make rounds at 9AM each morning, Monday through Friday. I expect you to be there with the rest of the staff. We meet in the room off the day room. Rounds usually last about two hours, and we go through all the orders on all the patients, keep the records current and deal with any important developments. In spite of your run-in with Bobbie, you will be relieved to know that you will not be doing electroshock on patients, though I may want you to observe or assist in the procedure from time to time.

Orders for patients usually go through me, unless some emergent issue comes up which will not wait, or when you are on night call. I do not care for new and innovative 'touchy-feely' therapies. We use a lot of medicines here and sometimes seclusion when things get out of hand.

Each afternoon after lunch we have a community meeting in the large day room, so that patients can air their concerns or grievances. Generally, it allows for some ventilation within reason to help keep the tone of frustration down. Your job is mainly to work up new arrivals, to help keep the records up to date, and to contribute any helpful information or insights that you might come up with. Any questions?"

"Not at this time, sir. If I think of anything, I'll get back to you."

"You can always check with Sadie, the head nurse. She is very well up on the routines around here if I am not readily available."

Quimby got up to leave but realized that he had not yet discussed the seminars that he was obliged to attend down at the University Hospitals across town.

"Dr. Nolan, I forgot to mention the seminars downtown."

"I know, every afternoon from 3 to 5 PM. You'll have to leave by 2:30, so I expect you will have your work completed prior to leaving. The nights that you are on call you will be expected to be back here on campus by 6PM. The on-call room is in the administrative building. The on- call list is in the information packet that you should have received. Night call is not usually onerous. Oh yes, one other thing. I do not approve of love affairs among the staff. They tend to be disruptive. Good luck, Quimby."

Fred left Dr. Nolan's office with some sense of relief. The chief's manner was rather brusque, and obviously he was a no-nonsense sort of leader.

Chapter three:
SEMINARS

Fred headed downtown to the main University campus where he was to meet with the other residents in his class and where he was to attend his first daily seminar. The seminar topics were to vary between psychological theories, medications and their management, looking at a variety of psychological testing procedures and their efficacy, and some time looking at both the theories and the history of Sigmund Freud and his followers and detractors. There was also a sort of group therapy where the residents could talk about their experiences with patients and how they handled them and how the experience affected them. Most important he would have the opportunity to compare notes with his colleagues who were in the same boat that he was.

When he entered the room, he was greeted by nine other residents, five males and four females. They introduced themselves and got acquainted. Though he had trouble remembering all the names, a few stood out. Two were older and had practiced as family doctors for a number of years before coming back to study psychiatry. One was a rather nervous Viet Nam war vet who had served as a combat physician and had clearly not left all the battles behind him. One was a gorgeous and clearly self-assured woman who had a great smile and seemed quite approachable, by the right guy. The others chattered among themselves until the instructor arrived and took control of the class. Fred tried to pay attention while the instructor went through the syllabus, but he kept glancing at the young beauty he had been introduced to as Miranda. She was about 5'5" with a smile that would stop a train. He hoped that she, too, was assigned across town at the state hospital, so he would have the opportunity to run into her there. It happens that he was in luck, and she was assigned to ward 2W, across the hall. He carefully and unobtrusively examined her left hand to make sure she was not wearing an engagement or wedding ring, and the finger being bare, Fred struck up a brief conversation with her after the instructor departed. He left hoping they might meet up sometime at the hospital cafeteria. Quimby was clearly interested in pursuing this woman.

It had been six years since his wife had died. Fred had married the love of his young life just after graduating from college and being accepted to medical school. They were very happy together as he entered medical school. Her parents had enough financial resources to help them manage through what could have been tough times. She worked some, but he was too occupied with his studies to contribute financially except through student loans. When she developed leukemia and quickly began to deteriorate, Fred was devastated. He dropped out of medical school, and when she died, he felt lost for about a year. Eventually he reapplied to the same school, and given his circumstances, was accepted back in. He managed to get his diploma, did his internship, and applied to a psychiatry program. He remembered his mother, who grew up in hard times and had to give up some of her dreams, saying, "Life is what goes on around you while you're planning other things." It was only recently that he felt that he could move on and could consider the idea of finding another woman that he could share love with.

The residents spent the rest of the afternoon getting acquainted with one another, chatting about their various backgrounds, looking at the upcoming content of the seminars, and essentially feeling each other out and registering first impressions. The schedule for the upcoming seminars were passed out.

They broke up about five o'clock, and some of the group went across the street to have a beer and get better acquainted. Fred joined them, especially when he saw that Miriam, the attractive young woman that piqued his interest, was planning to join them. They entered the bar, which was a college hangout, and it became obvious rather quickly that he was not the only one who was showing an interest in this sparkling resident. He did get an opportunity to spend a little time with her in conversation, but after about half an hour and two glasses of beer, he decided to call it a day, said 'adios' to the group, and headed out the door.

Chapter four: CLARENCE

Quimby had had the opportunity to get acquainted with the routines on the ward for a few days when his first new patient arrived. Clarence was a nerdy-looking man of about thirty years of age who was transferred from another hospital in a rural city about fifty miles distant. The patient was quite sunburned about his head and neck and ankles where he had been exposed to the sun for several days. He had climbed a water tower at the previous hospital and refused to come down, but eventually did so when he got thirsty and hungry and was convinced to get treatment for his sunburn. Fred showed him into his office to do the initial interview and exam. Clarence was quite meek and glanced around suspiciously. When Quimby asked him about the water tower incident, Clarence was at first reticent to talk about it, but then decided that he felt safe enough in this hospital to do so.

"I was worried because they were beginning to talk about releasing me, and once the mafia heard that, it would be all over for me. I decided that the only safe course for me would be to act crazy enough that they could not release me, and the mafia would then know that no one would believe my story."

"So, what was your story?" Fred asked.

"I really can't tell you that or we would both be in danger again."

"So, you know something that could put someone away?"

"Well, I really don't know anything, but they think I do."

"So, you think, that they think, that you know something that you really don't know, but if you did know, it would be dangerous because it could put someone in the mafia in prison?"

"Or on death row."

"But you don't know."

"But they think I do."

"And why do they think you do?"

"I really don't know."

"Maybe they are not really interested in you if you don't even know what it is that they think you know."

"No, I know it's true. Do you think I would spend three days and nights on a water tower getting sunburned and almost dying of thirst if it weren't true?"

This conversation was going in circles, and Quimby had to remind himself that this was a man whose thought process was not working normally, so he decided to get on with the rest of the workup and write up his findings. It happened that Clarence was from a poor family of Norwegian stock who finished high school and took an interest in becoming an amateur magician, entertaining at children's parties as a sideline from his other job as a gas station attendant. It was after one of these birthday party gigs at a wealthy Italian family's home that he became concerned about the mafia. The father of the family was influential in the community, and Clarence began to be convinced that he was "connected". It was downhill from there. Clarence was reluctant to do any more party gigs, and he became so fearful that he would not show up for work at the gas station and was fired. He spent all his time in his room until his parents, with whom he lived, had him hospitalized. The rest was history.

Just as Quimby was about to finish up and send Clarence back out to the unit, the new patient looked at Fred and said, "You look Italian. Are you Italian?"

It caught Quimby by surprise, and as he started to reply, "Well, ---"

Clarence jumped up, grabbed Fred, and started to wrestle with him. Fred was in that situation that he had been concerned about on that first day in his new office when he had fallen on his prat and no one had heard or come to his rescue.

On the floor, under the surprisingly wiry Clarence, Quimby said, "Clarence, I am a doctor not a member of the mafia. I am here to help you."

Something in his voice convinced Clarence to stop, get up off Quimby, help him up and to apologize. Fred straightened himself up, and gently showed Clarence to the door. Just as he was about to go out the door, Clarence turned and held out Fred's keys.

"Here, I had better return these to you. Again, I am sorry."

In the excitement, Quimby had not felt his pocket being picked by the amateur magician. He quickly checked for his wallet and was relieved that it was still there. He glanced at his wrist to check the time and realized his watch was gone.

"Clarence, what about my watch?"

"It's on your desk, Dr. Quimby." And it was – just lying there.

Chapter five:
ON CALL

It was Quimby's first night on call. Someone else was on for the weekend, but Fred had agreed to take Friday night for him, because the man had a previous commitment. Fred decided to be a good guy and help the guy out. The evening had been rather busy, mainly going from ward to ward filling out medication orders and weekend pass prescriptions that the service chiefs and residents had failed to take care of before scuttling off the units for the weekend. By about 10 PM he was back in the on-call room, had watched the evening news, and decided to hit the shower and go to bed. The warm shower felt good; he dried off and just crawled into the sheets, assuming that the rest of the night would be slow. The phone was nearby in case he was called, and his clothes were ready to jump into should he need to do so.

Fred had slept deeply for about an hour when he was jostled awake by movement and a woman's voice.

"Dr. Johnson?"

Sleepily, Fred answered, "No, it's Quimby. I took Johnson's call tonight."

The woman answered back. "That's OK, I'll settle for Quimby's Johnson." He recognized nurse Wanda's voice as she crawled into bed with him. She was as naked as he was.

She reached between his legs, and in a moment Fred was erect. Wanda swung her leg over him as if she were hopping onto a saddled horse, quickly positioned herself and directing Quimby's member into her, thrusting down. Quimby did not take long to react with an orgasm, but Wanda continued to thrust for several more minutes until she quivered, stiffened, made some muffled sounds and relaxed. She disengaged and swung her leg back over and lay next to the still surprised Quimby. She spoke first.

"Sorry if that was a little hurried for you, but I don't have to report to the unit until seven, so we'll be able to make that rooster crow again in a while. We'll take our time and enjoy it even more."

However, Quimby woke a little later to find Wanda gone. She was there and then she was gone. He wondered briefly if it had not all been a pubescent wet dream. He couldn't say he didn't enjoy it, but he wondered about the implications. He knew that he did not want Dr. Nolan to get word of this. Nor did he want any rumors to start that might complicate any chance he might have with Miranda. Wanda had obviously thought she was coming to have sex with Dr. Johnson but seemed to be not all that particular when she found out she was naked in bed with him. He hoped she would be discreet.

Chapter 6:
BACK ON THE WARD

Quimby walked somewhat bleary-eyed back onto the unit. He was still a bit rattled about the events of the night before. Quimby had settled on psychiatry as a career rather than any other medical specialty because it had seemed fascinating. He enjoyed talking to people but did not especially like "small talk" such as at cocktail parties, and psychiatry really got to the meat of things in people's lives as he saw it. It was also fascinating to think of turning the tables on some of the crazy notions that some patients might have. He remembered reading about one psychiatrist who worked at a large state hospital, where there was a patient who thought he was Jesus. The man was forever preaching, interfering with the therapy of others, and generally making a nuisance of himself because of his sincere efforts to save others. The doctor approached him one day and said, "I understand you know something about carpentry." Because he believed he was Jesus, who was raised by Joseph the carpenter, he paused and said, "Yes, I guess I do." The doctor then said, "Good, we need some help over at the carpentry shop, and I am sending you over there to give a hand." After several months of manual labor and working with wood, the patient began to settle into a more realistic existence and gradually emerged from his psychosis. Things like this fascinated Quimby, but he, himself, had to contend with the normal complexities of just living in the world. Last night was a bit bewildering. He really didn't know what to make of it.

He was still on duty until Dr. Johnson took over at noon. He had already been to the other wards for brief reports at the nursing stations and things were rather quiet. There were no rounds scheduled on the weekend. Wanda was the weekend nurse on this unit. When Fred looked at her, she had just a whisper of a smile. Otherwise, it was business as usual. And yes, last night he would have to live with, make sense of, and manage the results. He would just have to let "chronotherapy" do its work, i.e. let time pass and see what will come of it. He knew that Johnson was to relieve him, but he decided to keep the events of the evening to himself. He did not want to disrupt any ongoing relationship between Wanda and Dr. Johnson any more than his nocturnal encounter might have already done.

Fred had some time to kill until he was relieved, so he thought he would get to know some of the patients a bit better. He decided to get better acquainted with Wilfred Donne, "the poet". His Lewis Carroll quotation prior to meeting Dr. Nolan seemed to be quite prophetic. Before directing the patient into his office this time, he checked with Wanda as to whether Mr. Donne had ever been assaultive to anyone on the staff. The answer was a negative, so Fred decided it was safe to proceed.

As soon as they got into Fred's office, Mr. Donne began to quote poetry.

> "slipping your shirt down onto my skin
> I inhale your scent
> and close my eyes
> I feel you
> the softness of the fabric
> caressing my bare skin
> so sensual
> your scent enmeshing with mine
> lingering around me
> enveloping me
> in a hug
> that lasts all day
> wrapped in your essence
> when I can't be in your arms"

Quimby was startled. Was this guy picking up on the scent of his encounter with Wanda? He had planned to move on to something else by asking the patient about his history, where he had grown up, what his education was, what his home life had been like, and how he ended up in the hospital. However, before Quimby could open his mouth, the poet looked at him and said, "Glory be to God for dappled things—"

Quimby instinctively followed with, "For skies as couple-colored as a brindled cow;"

Coming back, the poet replied, "For rose-moles all in stipple upon trout that swim;"

And Quimby – "Fresh fire-coal chestnut-falls; finches wings;"

Back and forth they alternated lines of G.M. Hopkins poem, "Pied Beauty" to its last line. Fortunately, it was only eleven lines long, and Quimby was grateful for the interest he had taken in his literature courses in college.

Donne: "Know any Henley?"

Quimby: "Just the last stanza of Invictus –

It matters not how strait the gate,

How charged with punishments the scroll,

I am master of my fate;

I am the captain of my soul."

Donne: "I would have liked to have had you in my class."

Quimby: "I think I would have liked that."

Professor Donne closed his eyes, sat quietly for a moment, then said, "That's enough for today. I'll think about you for a while." He then got up and walked out the door of Fred's office.

Fred was dazed. He was trained as a physician, someone who managed the lives of others and who was supposed to maintain control. The last 24 hours had proved to him that his notion of being in control was going to change, that being in control in this business was going to have to be by recognizing that he could not control others or circumstances. He would have to learn to see the humor in this to survive in this field and to provide any help to others. He would just have to put some of his medical training and indoctrination aside and learn to go with the flow of his instincts.

Chapter 7:
HOSPITAL CAFETERIA

A week had gone by and Fred had seen little of Miranda other than briefly at seminars, but he struck a bit of luck when he went to the cafeteria for lunch. She was at a table by herself. Just as he got food for his tray and started to walk over to join her, Richard Johnson, the resident for whom he had taken the bewildering night call, pulled up a chair beside her. They seemed to be quite friendly, as if they were already well acquainted. Fred was crestfallen but did not want to show it. He walked over to their table and asked, "Mind if I join you?" Johnson pointed to a chair; Miranda appeared entranced with the debonair Dr. Johnson. They chatted about ward politics, patients, various encounters, their interests, but it was clear that those topics were secondary. They were noticeably interested in each other's company, and Fred felt like a fifth wheel. They needed him there like a fish needs a bicycle. Fred ate his lunch quickly and excused himself to get back to the ward, fuming inside about why he had been so worried about stepping on toes between Wanda and Johnson. It frustrated him to know that Johnson had been carrying on with Wanda and now seemed to have dropped her to carry on with Miranda, or maybe both. Yet Fred knew that he had no right to be angry, since he also had carried on with Wanda, albeit only the one time, at least so far. He still had to contend with the next time he would be on call, and what would happen if she showed up again.

When Fred got back to the ward, Wanda had a request for him. Apparently, a field trip had been planned with several of the well-behaved patients to go to the local historical museum. Clarence was on the list, but she needed permission to let him go on the accompanied trip because of the circumstances that had brought him to this hospital. Dr. Nolan was not in his office. He had been called for a conference to the State Offices. Sadie, the head nurse was also gone from the unit for the rest of the afternoon, so Wanda needed Fred's permission to let Clarence go, and Clarence had been on his best behavior since his arrival at the hospital. Wanda was sure that it would be allowable, but she needed a doctor's permission and asked Fred to allow it. Fred looked at Wanda and, without hesitation, signed the permission sheet. Meanwhile, Fred had a new patient waiting to be worked up. It was a young man with a rather glazed look about him who announced, "Hi doc, you are looking at a star-crossed lover, and I'm going to need your help."

This young man, named Lester Pickins, was led into Fred's office. He proceeded to tell Fred about his relationship with another young woman whom he had met on a field trip with his college class and with whom he had been sitting one evening when an exceptionally bright star erupted in the sky. He knew at that moment that they were meant to be together as "star-crossed lovers". When he mentioned this to her, she was obviously wary about him, but he did not understand why she should be, considering the celestial sign. He continued to pursue her, though she tried to ignore him. He took a picture of himself, poked pinholes in the eyes, shined a light behind the picture, then took a photo of the altered picture to look like his picture was emitting light from his eyes. He then sent it to her. He became fascinated with eyes and attempted to get into optometry school but was not accepted into the program. He continued to pursue the woman, but eventually the young woman got the police involved, and he ended up in the hospital. When Fred suggested to him that this behavior sounded crazy to a lot of people, and particularly to this young woman, and I questioned why he persisted in this pursuit. His response was, "Doc, if I give this up, then I would just be a nobody. Look at my eyes. Can't you see that this is real and meant to be?"

Once again, Quimby had to admit to himself that a lot of distorted thinking occurs as a human response, often out of fear or loneliness. Fred finished up his workup and excused Lester back to the ward. He wrote up his initial findings of a delusional disorder, but something about Lester was haunting, and it bothered him. He realized that his own loss was part of it. He had been in an idyllic state after his marriage. They planned to have children, settle into a regular routine and raise a family as their parents had done. That was a dream that would not come true, and he could profoundly appreciate the loss of love that Lester felt, even though it was delusional.

Chapter 8:
END OF THE WORK DAY

It was close to 5:00 and there was no seminar this day, so Fred left the hospital and walked to the parking lot trying to remember where he had parked. He scanned the lot and saw the red-dyed tennis ball on the top of the aerial of his seven-year-old Chevy, walked over to it and got in. On the ride to his apartment, his back door suddenly opened and out jumped Rudy with the car going about twenty-five miles per hour. Seeing Rudy rolling in the street. Fred screeched to a stop and ran to Rudy, who looked dazed.

"Rudy, what are you doing in my car?"

"I just had to get out of there. I can't live like this." was the reply.

Fortunately, Fred spotted a police car parked nearby, probably there to spot speeders. He ran over to the policeman and explained that Rudy was a patient at the State Hospital who had "eloped" and needed to get back to his unit. The policeman called for help and Fred waited with Rudy until he could be taken to the local ER for a medical checkup before being sent back to 2E. Fred asked,

"Rudy, how did you get into my car? It was locked."

"I have a friend who taught me how to pick locks and to break into cars.", was his reply.

Fred breathed a sigh and proceeded to stop for a quick hamburger and fries before going to his apartment. It was almost nine that evening by the time he got home to his 2-bedroom place. He had converted one bedroom to a sort of study where he had a small desk and some bookcases. The living room had some garage sale furniture and a TV. The kitchen was a nook with a stove and frig and a set of cabinets. It could have been cozy, but it was bland – mainly a place to crash. Fred sat on the couch and picked up an anthology of poetry, but he was too tired to read, so he turned on the TV. Nothing much was on, and he dozed.

It must have been about 3AM when a knock at the door awakened him. The TV was still on. He shut it off and went to the door. Standing at the entrance to his apartment was none other than Clarence, with a desperate look on his face and a sword in his hand.

Needless to say Fred was startled. "Clarence, what in hell are you doing here at this time of night? What are you doing with that sword? What's going on? Why aren't you at the hospital?"

Clarence stuttered something about the mafia, about defending himself, and coming to Fred for safety. He had been on the outing to the historical society museum and had gotten fearful and slipped away and hid himself under one of the hoop skirts of the display mannequins. He hid there all day until closing time and then crept out to find a telephone, which he hoped he could use to call the FBI. He realized however, that at this time of night he would not be able to reach any of the agents, so he decided to call long distance to the New York Times to talk to a reporter about his fears. The reporter apparently kept him on the line long enough to trace the call and notify the local police. When Clarence saw flashing lights through a window, he grabbed a display sword and scooted out the back door.

"And how did you find my place? I'm not listed in the phone book."

"I might be considered crazy by some, but I am intelligent, Dr. Quimby. I have my ways of finding things."

"Why the sword, Clarence? Did you plan to hurt someone?"

"No, just insurance for protection. I took up fencing in the short time that I attended college. I was pretty good at it."

He did a quick demonstration of his agility with the rapier which both impressed and intimidated Quimby, who was grateful that Clarence no longer associated his being of Italian descent with being in the mafia.

"We've got to get you back to the hospital pronto, Clarence. And I have to get this sword back to the historical museum first thing in the morning."

Clarence would not allow Fred to call the police. He insisted that Fred take him back to the hospital himself and made such a fuss about it that, at 4AM, they arrived at 2E bleary-eyed. Clarence was hustled off to his room while Fred found a safe place to deposit the sword.

Fred noticed that there was a new admission for him to work up the next day and knew it would be a long one with the meager rest he had gotten that night with the adventures of Rudy and Clarence.

Chapter 9:
REPERCUSSIONS

After a couple of hours of much-needed but inadequate sleep, Quimby arrived at 2E to start another day. As he walked into the nursing station to check in, he was greeted apologetically by Wanda who handed him a note from Dr. Nolan who wanted to see him as soon as he arrived on the unit. He quickly complied and walked to the boss's office. Upon entering, he was met with what to Fred was a glaring snarl.

"And just what the hell were you up to yesterday in my absence, Quimby?"

"I must admit that I had quite a night, Dr. Nolan."

"Whose idea was it to let that Jensen patient go with the group to the historical museum?"

Fred did not want to get Wanda into trouble for bringing it up, so he took the heat himself.

"Clarence has been a model patient since he's been here, Dr. Nolan. You were gone, so I looked at his record and said to myself, what would Dr. Nolan do in this situation? Having observed you making various decisions over the last several weeks, I said to myself, it is well-supervised, and I think Dr. Nolan would let him go, so I agreed to do so."

"And that other rascal, Rudy? What was that all about? He is always pulling some shenanigans, half the time trying to get himself killed."

"Well, you know Rudy. He unfortunately is pretty smart and somehow managed to find my car in the lot and get into it even though I had locked it. He hid in it until I left the hospital property and then jumped out while I was driving. It's fortunate I had slowed down enough when I heard the door open that he wasn't badly hurt. I did manage to hail a cop to get him to the ER and then back to the hospital. All in all, I was very lucky to get both of those rascals back to the hospital safely without any major injuries or incidents. Yes, sir, it was quite a night. I hope you are satisfied with the eventual outcome."

"No major incidents? Jensen stole a valuable sword and called a major newspaper with a story that could put this hospital on the map as a laughing stock. Then he shows up at a doctor's residence with the sword. That's not a major incident?"

"Well, sir, no one was injured other than Rudy's minor scrapes and bruises, and the Clarence situation was handled without getting the police involved, other than getting the sword back to where it belongs, which I will make sure happens in a timely fashion."

Dr. Nolan seemed to calm down. He sat there awhile and then had the where-with-all to take a breath, let it out, and then to take stock of Quimby's summary of the situation. He seemed relieved and said, "Quimby, it looks like you handled both situations quite well professionally. You kept your head and saved me some grief. Thanks, that's all for now."

Fred quickly exited the office, also breathing a sigh of relief.

Fred's next task was to make sure the sword got back to the museum. He went to the nursing station where he had stashed it and made arrangements to get it transported back to town by one of the orderlies who was about to go off duty. The orderly was not to mention the hospital, but to tell the museum staff that he had found it on the grounds outside the museum. That, hopefully, would keep some of the hubbub about the hospital field trip to a minimum.

Fred's next step was to have a sit-down with Clarence to get up-dated on just what did happen while he was at the museum and why. He asked that Clarence be awakened and sent to his office, so he could go over the events of yesterday with him.

When Clarence entered the office, he was understandably as bleary-eyed as Fred.

Fred sat awhile looking at Clarence before asking, "OK, Clarence, why the New York Times?"

"Because it's motto is 'All the news that's fit to print'." was the reply.

Fred, puzzled, shook his head and said, "What kind of answer is that?"

Clarence was somewhat bewildered that Dr. Quimby did not understand. He said that he became quite frightened that his cover might be blown and decided to call the NY Times. He knew that if the information that he knew came out from there, it was too big an organization for the mafia to control, and he would not be in such danger. They would not dare to come after him without revealing that they were the guilty ones.

"We've been over this before, Dr. Q."

"So, Clarence, what did you tell the people at the Times?"

"I cannot tell you that, Dr. Quimby, until they come out with it in their paper, in which case you can just read about it, and I won't have to tell you. I don't want to put you in any danger."

"So this is another 'Catch 22' is it, Clarence? You cannot tell me, but if the truth comes out, you don't have to. You told me the last time we talked that you really didn't know anything, that they just think that you do."

"That's about it, Doc, but just because I don't know anything doesn't mean that the newspaper won't investigate." he sheepishly replied.

"You have a propensity for dramatic flourishes, Clarence, first the water tower, and now this. Please ease off, my friend."

"Well thank you, Dr. Q. I am beginning to feel like we are becoming friends when we have talks like this. You tend to be very understanding. By the way, here are your keys. I believe you misplaced them again." Clarence handed Quimby his key ring with the keys to his car and apartment.

Quimby was astounded but tried to keep his surprise and frustration to himself. He thanked Clarence and then excused him. Fred remembered he had yet another task. Although he was really tired, but he had another new patient waiting to be seen that morning.

Chapter 10:
ANOTHER NEW EXPERIENCE

Fred knew he had work to do before leaving for his afternoon seminars. He went to the nursing station to find his new patient and located his chart. The young man's name was Jonathon Maxwell. He was able to find him on the unit, introduced himself, and led the young man to his office. As he did so, he heard Professor Donne intoning a part of Eliot's poem "The Hollow Men" in a low voice.

"Between the idea
And the reality
Between the motion
And the act
Falls the Shadow"

Fred wasn't sure what the poet, as he was often referred to, was picking up on, but he made a mental note of it.

The patient was relatively young and shy. Fred started his routine assessment and asked him his name. The reply came in a quiet high voice.

"Peter."

"Is that your middle name?" Quimby asked.

"No, I'm Peter." Came the reply in a very child-like voice.

"How old are you, Peter?" queried Quimby.

"Five." Was the reply.

Quimby looked a bit puzzled, wondering momentarily if he had the wrong patient, but, after he looked at the patient chart and saw a picture of the individual on the first page, he knew he had it right. He looked at some of the referral information and saw that this young man had been picked up by the police wandering and looking lost. When the police began to talk to him, he had suddenly become obstreperous and belligerent, changing his posture and demeanor rapidly. He had been put on a police-hold and brought to the hospital where he was admitted to a psychiatric unit. Within a short time, he had become reasonable and, in a hearing before the judge, apologized profusely, so he was released with the recommendation that he seek outpatient treatment. Several other incidents like this resulted in his eventual commitment to this hospital. Quimby suspected a dissociative disorder. He thought for a moment and asked the patient, "Could I please speak to Jonathon? It is very important."

The child-like person in front of him, paused, lowered his head for a moment, and then raised his head again and, in a lower voice said, "Hello, I'm Jonathon. How can I help you?"

Fred suddenly realized that the poet had nailed it again. The man had an uncanny knack for picking up on subtleties on this unit. This new patient clearly had what was called a multiple personality disorder, experiencing various personalities that would show up in different circumstances and situations as a defense mechanism to protect him, depending on what and how he perceived them as threatening. The child personality was like the puppy who rolled over on his back with bigger dogs to show subservience, like saying, "I'm just a puppy. Don't hurt me." The Jonathon personality was the day-to-day take care of business part of him. Often there would be other parts that would come out depending on whether physical fighting was thought to be necessary, or just spiteful behavior arising out of anger and frustration. Often these alternate personalities, or "alters", were not all aware of each other. This patient would take a lot of time to get to know.

Fred got the basic information that he needed for the initial workup, but he knew that he had much more to learn about this young man. Meanwhile, he had a seminar to get to.

Chapter 11:
DISENCHANTMENT AND MORE

The seminar topic was "Delusions and Humor and how to interpose the two in the treatment process". For Fred, it was not humorous to see Miranda and Dick Johnson being so cozy and friendly during the presentation, even though the content of the meeting was pertinent to some of what he had to contend with on 2E. After the meeting, Fred watched the two depart together with a lingering feeling of disappointment. The worst of all was Johnson's query to Quimby about how he was getting along with "that good looking redhead, Wanda on 2E". It galled him that the guy had obviously been intimate with her before Fred had, and now he was busily engaged with pursuing Miranda. At the same time, he also recognized his own envy over the fact that he was not in the stellar position with Miranda that Johnson was.

Fred left the seminar alone and wandered to a local bar called The Brewhouse. He sat at the bar, ordered a draft beer, and started to sip it and watch the local news on TV when he felt a tap on his shoulder. He turned to look into the eyes of Wanda. He started to say something to her, but she put her fingers on his lips and said, "Shhhh, don't say anything until I apologize to you. Let's go find a table where we can talk."

They went to a quiet corner and sat down. Wanda told him that she was very glad that he had come in, because she had hoped to find a place away from work where she could tell him how sorry she was for putting him in a compromising and perhaps embarrassing position.

"As you can probably guess, I have known Dick Johnson for a while. We went to high school together and I had a crush on him for a long time. We ended up years later, I, a nurse and he a doctor, at the same hospital, and when he, suddenly took an interest in me, I was thrilled. We had a short sexual affair and when he asked me to rendezvous with him in the on-call room, I was a little nervous about doing it at work, but I agreed. Little did I know that he had set up both of us.

When I climbed in bed with you and realized what he had done, I decided to go ahead and have sex with you. I would tell him about how great it was and make him jealous, but I quickly realized that it had been a mistake. So, in spite of the fact that I really had enjoyed it with you, that is why I left as soon as you fell asleep. I am sorry if I put you in a bad situation. I am sorry that I treated you disrespectfully. I have seen you as a good guy working on our unit, and I am truly sorry for appearing so distant and callous and for putting you in a tenuous situation."

Quimby looked at the tears starting to well in her eyes and reached out to touch her hand.

"I cannot say I was disappointed with what happened. I was quite surprised, but pleasantly so. I was confused with how it all came about and by your abrupt departure. I didn't know what to make of it all, but I did enjoy our encounter. I had not had sex for quite a while since my wife had died, and I have missed that kind of intimate connection. I have no regrets about our time alone together. I am sorry if it caused you pain or embarrassment. Please don't worry about me. I am OK. The question is, how are you?"

"You are a kind man, Fred Quimby. I hope you can forgive me."

"Forgive you? I would like to take you out to dinner and a movie sometime, as long as we don't let old man Nolan know about it. It would just be a date. I would not be expecting to make it another bedtime story."

"I have to give that a little time to sink in, but thank you. I'll see you at work. I do want to let you know that I am grateful that you took the heat for the Clarence debacle. I am sure that Dr. Nolan got on your case about that."

"It all worked out OK. I managed to cool old Nolan down a bit. He seemed to feel it turned out all right. Don't worry about it. I'm glad we had a chance to talk. I'll see you soon."

Fred watched her walk out of the bar feeling a bit sad for her, but he also felt a twinge of a thrill.

Chapter 12:
A SUNDAY ON THE WARD
August 1969

The patients on 2E often found weekends to be boring. Routines were less regimented, and patients felt they had more leisure time to read, play cards, write letters, or whatever else they could find to amuse themselves, but it also left them more time to be alone with their thoughts. On this particular Sunday morning, Clarence approached Wilfred Donne as he sat in the dayroom reading, sat down next to him, and handed him a note. On it was written: "In your room under your mattress is a copy of the book that was taken from you when you entered the hospital."

Donne looked at him and said, "How do you know about that book?"

Clarence replied, "You don't need to know the particulars. I just wanted to help a fellow traveler." He then got up and wandered out of the dayroom.

Wilfred sat for a while, looked around to see if anyone had been watching them, and slowly got up to go to his room. The book was under the mattress. It was Wilfred's handwritten journal. Apparently, the staff or the doctors thought it would impede his progress and did not want him to focus on the issues that had led him to his present state of mind. The "poet" assumed they had probably destroyed it, and that thought crushed his spirit, since a lot of his musings, thoughts and reflections had gone into that journal. It was the one activity that he felt had helped him hold on to his sanity. Somehow, Lord knows how, Clarence had managed to get his hands on it and rescue it for him.

He had watched Clarence on the ward and thought that he had been suitably placed in the hospital, but suddenly he had a warm feeling toward this Robin Hood character. Wilfred pondered the situation for a while. He had observed the rather stealthy approach that this character Clarence took to most things on the unit. He then quickly penned a note, quoting Robert Frost's poem, In Neglect:

> *"They leave us so to the way we took,*
> *As two to whom they were proved mistaken,*
> *That we sit sometimes in the wayside nook,*
> *With mischievous, vagrant, seraphic look,*
> *And try if we cannot feel forsaken."*

When Clarence read this note a bit later, he thought it a bit obtuse, but he knew he had made a friend and one who was smart enough to be helpful if necessary.

At lunchtime Wilfred seated himself at the same table with Clarence. To an astute observer, this would have appeared a bit unusual, since both were usually solitary eaters. Clarence spoke first.

"People think I'm nuts because I worry about the people that I used to work for, who are Italian, and I suspect, are relatively high up in the mafioso."

Wilfred looked at him long and hard before answering, "I know. People think I'm nuts because I quit my job after my wife split with a low-life, and I chose to retreat into things that I loved, books and ideas. And here we are, stuck in this place."

"Well," Clarence retorted, "at least it's safe here."

Wilfred frowned. "Safe from freedom? What then?"

After a pause, "By the way, how did you manage to come up with my journal?"

Clarence smiled and said, "I worked for some time as an amateur magician, and in the process, I learned to distract people enough to pick their pockets or take things by diverting their attention. I managed to take the keys to the storage area from the head nurse long enough to get into it before returning the key. Your journal was pretty easy to find."

Wilfred stroked the stubble on his chin. He backed off his tendency to quote poetry to make his feelings known and just said, "Thanks, Clarence. Having that book back has given me a sense of self-ownership again. I haven't had that since I arrived here. If you ever need something that I can help with, I'm in your corner."

Clarence tipped his head down and said, "Thanks, Wilfred, I haven't felt like I've had someone I could count on since I got here. I appreciate that."

They finished their lunch and ate their pudding dessert in silence, both clearly less anxious and looking rather content. This Sunday turned out to be better than most.

Chapter 13:
MONDAY ON THE WARD AGAIN

Morning rounds were over and for once no new patients had arrived over the weekend to work up. Fred pondered whether he should spend time with the patient with the dissociative disorder, Jonathon, or whether he should check in on Clarence or Wilfred. He was walking toward Jonathon when Wilfred approached him.

"Might I have a word with you Dr. Quimby?"

"Of course, Mr. Donne. What's on your mind?"

"Can we talk privately in your office?"

"Yes, we can. I would be happy to. Let's saunter down this way."

They walked down the hall to Quimby's office. He unlocked the door and followed Wilfred in. Fred always had an emotional memory of the time he had been accosted by Clarence in this room. He had since moved the furniture so that his chair was now closest to the door. He motioned Wilfred to have a seat, and he did likewise.

"What's on your mind, Mr. Donne?"

"I've been here a number of months, and I've been thinking a lot about things. I've wondered what it is that I need to do to get discharged from this place. I think I am quite alert. I have just had a lot on my mind and had trouble shaking it off."

Quimby thought about it. Here was a man who was quite astute, well-read, and educated, but who had had a significant blow to his ego – a blow that had left him staggered. Fred thought about the line from Milton's "Paradise Lost"

> *"Nine times the space that measures day and night*
> *To mortal men, he with his horrid crew*
> *Lay vanquished, rolling in the fiery gulf*
> *Confounded though immortal: But his doom*
> *Reserved him to more wrath; for now the thought*
> *Both of lost happiness and lasting pain*
> *Torments him:"*

The poem referred to Satan, but Wilfred had been seriously traumatized by the departure of his wife, and with her, his hopes for the future. What he had now were his books, his mind, but little hope for intimacy. He had no children, and his nuclear family was gone. Fred thought about taking a different tack with Wilfred.

"Wilfred, you have a significant library at home, don't you?"

"Well, yes, but what does that have to do with anything?"

"I would like you to think about a different library that you own. You have a library of your thoughts and experiences. Think of some of the stories that you have on those shelves – childhood memories, sports experiences, educational thrills, teenage dating, and many more, I am sure. Each of those books has a healing content that is available to you and can help you to move on past the rip tides, avalanches, and crevasses of your life to better things. Right now, you seem to be mired in a book titled, *Loss*. Maybe it's time to take another book off the shelf and open it."

Wilfred appeared startled. He had not thought about his life as a series of adventures and mishaps. He had not thought about his being and living in the context of his beloved books.

Suddenly there was the sound of a lot of running near the old drinking fountain on the unit, a loud "bonk" sound, and more noise as people crowded around someone lying on the floor. Fred opened the door to his office and ran over to find two aides tending to Rudy, who had run and taken a head-first dive into the ceramic fountain with a cast-iron spout. His head was bleeding, and he was unconscious on the floor. The spout on the fountain was quite bent. Rudy woke to a confused consciousness and said, "I'm sorry." An ambulance was called so that Rudy could be transported to the general hospital downtown to be treated for the head wound and checked for other damage. Another rather unusual and fortunately unsuccessful suicide attempt by Rudy. Another exciting day on the unit.

Fred looked around, scanning the unit for any emotional repercussions among the patients. Wilfred was gone. Clarence was watching with some apprehension from the other side of the day room. Fred decided to check on him and walked across the room.

Clarence said, "It's not even safe in here sometimes."

Fred said, "It's Okay, Clarence, we'll make sure he is taken care of and is safe."

Clarence shook his head and walked off toward his room.

Chapter 14:
A WEEK LATER

Quimby arrived on the unit to find that Clarence had been taken to the general hospital the day before. After Rudy's mishap he had apparently become so worried, that he began to fear being poisoned. He began drinking a lot of water, trying to dilute any poison that someone might put into his food. He carried water with him, sipping on it incessantly. Unfortunately, over a week's time, he managed to dilute his blood electrolytes so much that he became hyponatremic and had a seizure, requiring him to be shipped to another hospital to re-stabilize his sodium and potassium blood levels. Fred was met on the unit by Wilfred, who, to Fred's surprise, was visibly upset about Clarence's situation.

"Doc, can you please find out for me how Clarence is doing? Does he need a blood transfusion or anything? I'll be glad to donate if it would help."

Fred tried to reassure Wilfred that the hospital would be taking good care of Clarence and said he would find out about Clarence's condition as soon as he could and would get back to him. He was a bit surprised by the intensity of this new relationship, but he was happy to see Wilfred having a caring response about someone outside of himself.

Fred walked to the nursing station. Wanda was back from being gone for a week. Fred wondered whether she had been ill.

"Hello, good nurse, it's great to see you back. Are you feeling well?"

"Yes, I had a bit of a family crisis and took some time off, but everything turned out well in the long run."

"Anything you need? Anything I can help you with?"

"I think things are under control now, but I appreciate your asking."

"Tell you what – why don't we sit down over a cup of coffee after work and you can tell me about it, and if I can help in any way, I will."

Wanda hesitated, but it was clear that she was pulled by the idea of having someone she was inclined to trust offering to listen and give her the opportunity to sort things out. She liked Fred, though she was still embarrassed by their encounter in the on-call room.

She replied, "That's very nice. I'd like that. How about that little coffee shop near the campus around five?"

"Better yet," said Fred, "how about I take you out to dinner at that little steak house on River Street? We can relax and have a good meal while we're at it."

Wanda smiled and said, "OK, it's a deal. I'll meet you there after work."

Fred said, "OK then. After work it is." He felt rather exhilarated at the prospect of a date and was rather surprised at himself. His early infatuation with his co-resident, Miranda, had waned, especially since she seemed to be smitten by Dr. Johnson, whom he was increasingly growing to dislike.

Chapter 15:
THE STEAK HOUSE

Fred arrived before Wanda and found a table in a corner that was relatively private. He had learned a lot in the last several months, both professionally and privately. He had become more comfortable with his own spontaneity with patients and was surprised at his ability to follow his instincts. Today was one of those times. He looked forward to seeing Wanda and just having a friendly get-together with her. He realized that the sex with her was just a memorable accident, a pleasant one, but that he really liked her and was looking forward to her company.

As Fred glanced over the menu, he looked up and there was Wanda, hand in hand with a child of about 5-6 years – a cute little girl with red hair like Wanda's.

"Hi Fred, I took the liberty to bring along my daughter. I just picked her up from the sitter. Maria, this is Fred. Fred this is Maria."

"Well, how do you do, Maria. It is very nice to meet you. How old are you?"

"I am six years old. Are you really a doctor?"

"Well, yes I am, but I am not a shot doctor. I am a feelings doctor. Do you know what that is?"

"Do you help people with their feelings?"

"Yes, that's exactly what I do. Speaking of feelings, how do you feel about coming to a grownup place like this to have a nice dinner?"

Maria looked around and said, "It sure smells good."

Fred smiled and said, "Well let's look at the menu and see if we can find something to eat that will taste as good as it smells in here."

Wanda appeared to be pleased that this surprise encounter between Fred and Maria had started out so pleasantly. She had not been sure how this would sit with him, but she decided it was time for him to be aware of a little of her past before any potential relationship proceeded further.

The meal went well. Maria was able to enjoy "the best hamburger" she had so far eaten, along with garlic French fries and a few baked beans. The conversation was animated between Fred and Maria, and Wanda beamed throughout the meal. It was unspoken that Wanda and Fred would talk about this night on another occasion, and for now, they would just enjoy each other's company. When the meal was over, Fred picked up the tab, gave Maria a hug, and shook Wanda's hand.

"I'll see you tomorrow at work, Wanda. Thanks for introducing me to Maria and letting me spend a nice evening with you both."

Wanda smiled. "Thanks for dinner, Fred. We both had a great time."

Maria curtsied. "Thank you, Fred. It was very nice to meet you. I hope we can see you again soon."

"Let's make that a pinky promise, Maria." And he held out his little finger to grip hers as they both smiled.

The evening together was over, but the thoughts and feelings had just begun. Fred realized that Maria was just about the age his own child would have been had the original plans to have a child not been put on hold because of his wife's illness and subsequent death. Fred was not a religious man, but he could not put the thought out of his mind that perhaps his dead wife's spirit might be guiding him to and through a labyrinth of pathways to a happy life.

Chapter 16:
GROWING DESPERATION
October 1969

Wilfred Donne sat in the day room musing about his circumstances. His focus was on Chester, the brain-injured man who was staring out the window, then on Rudy pacing frantically, and back to the several patients looking blankly at the TV. Wilfred's mind drifted to the poem by Edwin Markham, "The Man with the Hoe".

"Bowed by the weight of centuries he leans
Upon his hoe and gazes on the ground,
The emptiness of ages on his face,
And on his back the burden of the world.
Who made him dead to rapture and despair,
A thing that grieves not and never hopes.
Stolid and stunned, a brother to the ox?
Who loosened and let down this brutal jaw?
Whose was the hand that slanted back this brow?
Whose breath blew out the light within this brain?"

Wilfred got up and left the day room. He felt the need to get out of this place. He had spent enough time grieving. It was time to get on with his newly discovered "library" so that he could reclaim his life and become happy, or at least comfortable with himself again. He looked for Clarence who was now back from the hospital downtown. He needed someone to talk to who, at least at times, seemed to make sense. Clarence was in his room sitting on his bed and staring at the wall.

"Clarence, we've got to get out of this place. It's deadening to us. It's stultifying! We have to find a way."

"It's no use for me, Wilfred. I'm afraid. It's too fearful for me out there. I'll be swallowed up and killed."

"We're dying day-by-day in here, Clarence. We have to learn to live. Out there we have a chance. You're not actually afraid of the mafia, are you? You're afraid of the world, and you really don't know what that even means, do you?"

"The mafia is something I can focus on."

"But for you that threat is not even real. You need a new set of glasses to view the world. Start sorting it out with Quimby. He can help you. He helped me. I know now that my time here is over, and I need to move on. And I may need your help. If I can't get them to discharge me, I know that you are clever enough and have the skills to help me escape."

With a stare from Clarence that went through to his bones, Wilfred backed up a bit and said, "OK, Clarence, please think about it. You're the only friend I really have in this place. I'd like to keep you as a friend, and I'd like good things for you as well."

Wilfred reached out gently and put his hand on the slumped shoulder of Clarence. He could see that his friend needed time to do his own sorting.

"I'll leave you alone, Clarence, but I want you to know that you have a friend in me, and I am willing to help you in any way that I can."

Wilfred got up and quietly walked to his own room. He found a pencil and paper and began to write.

The note read: "Clarence, I know that you are afraid. I've been afraid too. For some reason, Fred Quimby saw something in me that helped me see an alternative.

I came across an anonymous poem some time back that now suddenly made a lot of sense to me. I'll share it with you in hopes that it is also helpful to you. It's called *Fear*:

> 'It is said that before entering the sea
> a river trembles with fear.
> She looks back at the path she has traveled,
> from the peaks of the mountains,
> the long winding road crossing forests and villages.

*And in front of her,
she sees an ocean so vast,
that to enter
there seems nothing more than to
disappear forever.
But there is no other way.
The river cannot go back.
Nobody can go back.
To go back is impossible in existence.
The river needs to take the risk
of entering the ocean
because only then will fear disappear,
because that's where the river will know
it's not about disappearing into the ocean,
but of becoming the ocean.'*

Clarence, this is not meant to be a lecture. Lord knows I have given enough of those in the classroom. I would just like to have you accept this note as a gift from a friend as you have shown yourself to be to me."

Wilfred got up, walked to Clarence's room, and seeing that he had left the room, put the note under his pillow and left.

When Clarence found the note later, he opened and read it. He stared at it awhile. Tears filled his eyes. He softly said, "I thank you, my friend, but I'm just not ready for this quite yet; I'll keep it to remind me that I can count on you, and I'll help you with whatever I can."

Chapter 17:
MORE EXCITEMENT ON THE UNIT

When Fred walked into the unit on this particular morning, he heard loud voices coming from the dayroom. Everyone seemed to be congregated there. He rushed to see what was happening. Jonathon Maxwell was at one end of the room with people crowded around. He was wielding the broken off arm of a chair and threatening Wanda the nurse with it. Wilfred Dunne was nearby trying to talk to him in a calm voice.

Fred approached and spoke to Jonathon in a steady but firm voice, "Jonathon, I need you to focus on me."

"I'm not Jonathon!" he yelled back.

"Tell me your name." Fred spoke in a calm but firm voice.

"None of your business." Was the retort.

"I need to know your name, so I know to whom I am speaking." Fred was firm.

"I'm Jack. What's it to you?"

"Jack, I need to speak to the manager."

"Who are you talking about?"

"Jack, you know full well about whom I am referring. There are a number of individuals --- all taking turns ---coming out to take care of Jonathon. I want to speak to the organizer. I know you know his name. I want to speak to him or her, and I will introduce myself. In the meantime, you need to close your eyes, go to sleep, and stay asleep while the manager and I take care of business and keep the rest of you out of trouble. Now put your head down on your chest and go to sleep."

"Fuck you! I'm going to take care of business myself right now with this nurse. She's a busybody trying to boss me around, telling me to be quiet and leave the room."

"She's doing her job, Jack. She's just trying to keep you out of trouble. Now I know that all this excitement has made you tired. You look very, very, tired. I want you to calm down, put your chin on your chest, take some deep breaths, and let the tiredness close your eyes. You can even slip into a restful sleep until we can straighten this thing out. While you are sleeping, the manager and I will work out the details to try to keep you all out of trouble. That's right, just let your eyes let you go to sleep."

Jack seemed to be wrestling with that command within himself, but his lids began to sag, he put his chin on his chest and closed his eyes. He seemed to doze off. His eyes then reopened, and his countenance changed to a softer, quieter demeanor.

"Hello, Dr. Quimby, I am Randolph. How can I help you?"

"Randolph, I am glad to finally meet you. I've met Peter and Jonathon and now Jack. I think we need to talk about how to help me get to know the others, so that we together can coordinate this chamber orchestra to your advantage. So far it's been a little out of tune."

"I would like to talk a little more in private, Dr. Quimby. It's a bit crowded to talk about personal stuff here in the dayroom."

"Agreed, Randolph, but I want to remind Jack to continue his siesta until I give him permission to join us."

He turned to look at Wanda and gently asked, "Wanda, are you OK? Did Jack injure you?"

Wanda looked relieved that Fred had settled things down and nodded that she was OK.

Fred returned his attention to Randolph and said,

"Let's go to my office, Randolph, and see what we can do to make this a more workable relationship."

The day room went from a tense confrontation to calm conversation and patients and staff alike made room for Fred and Randolph to pass.

Once in Fred's office, Randolph seemed to develop a semblance of trust in Fred and was able to tell him about some of the machinations of the defensive system that had built up over time due to Jonathon's history of being in abusive situations.

Peter was the little boy personality that was like the little puppy that rolls over in submission to larger dogs. Jack was the aggressive, rebellious, fight-back teenage personality. Jonathon was often confused because of the fact that he was unaware of many of the others. He had periods of amnesia for events that occurred when other personalities presented themselves. Randolph rarely came out but was the cohesive part that tried to keep it all together and knew the other personalities and their patterns of behavior.

Fred was able to get Randolph to agree to put the names and idiosyncrasies of the other personalities down on paper. Fred was also able to stress the eventual need for all the personalities to become aware of each other, making it easier to communicate freely with one another. Fred reminded Randolph that they all share the same space and suffer the same consequences for whatever behavior any one of them does. They both agreed to meet again the next day to discuss things further, and Randolph left the office quietly.

Fred immediately went to the nurse's station to check on Wanda. She was rather calm outwardly, but it was a scary situation to be accosted by a patient with a club.

"Dr. Quimby, good job! That man was wound up for a good 15 minutes before you came in, and he was continuing to escalate. You calmed him down quickly."

"Well, the secret seemed to be getting his attention. But how are you? That had to be quite scary. I was worried about you. How are the rest of the people on the unit after all the hullabaloo?"

"Things are pretty calm. Once people saw that you had taken control of the situation, they settled down. Thanks again, Dr. Q."

"Well, got to get back to work. Excitement is over. I have other stuff to catch up on. I still have more work to do with this guy, but things should stay calm for now." Fred breathed a sigh of relief.

Fred understood that he would need all his skill and knowledge to be successful with Jonathon and his cohorts. He knew that people with multiple personality disorder were particularly susceptible to hypnotic suggestion. He hoped to keep Jack in a sleep mode for an extended time to keep that defensive part of the personality under control until other issues could be dealt with. He would use Randolph, the reasoning persona to gather enough information to get a further understanding of the traumas that Jonathon had experienced. He knew that he had to treat the various personalities, or "alters", as though they were a special kind of jigsaw puzzle. Until they all knew about the different pieces or parts of themselves and how they fit together, they would not be able to see how their total human picture worked. Treatment would be a long haul. Not only did the different alters have to become aware of each other, they would also have to accept each other and communicate to become one unit, one person, eventually.

Fred looked over at Wanda. "Join me for lunch today at the cafeteria?"

She winked at him and said, "Sounds good. See you there."

Fred wanted to check in with Wilfred. The poet had also been in the thick of the activity on the ward. He had been trying to calm Jack down to keep him from hurting Wanda. Fred and Wilfred also had not completed their conversation about the poet's discharge and how that might come about.

Fred found his way to the day room where he saw Wilfred gazing around at the other patients. Fred sat down next to him.

"Hello, Wilfred, may I talk with you? I wanted to check on you after all that excitement earlier. We also did not get to finish our conversation the other day when we were interrupted by the situation with Rudy."

"Doc, I need to get out of this place. Our conversation last time opened up my eyes to a number of things. I don't need to be here anymore. I'm ready to pick up my life and make it count again. You're a good doc. You connected with me so I could hear you and look at other options for myself. I saw how you handled that guy in the dayroom that no one else could calm down. I need you to help me do this right."

"Wilfred, you were ready to hear me. It wasn't just me. The timing was right. Your emotional growth brought you to that decision. What will you do when you get out of here? Do you have employment prospects, family, friends? Why don't you put a plan together so Dr. Nolan can justify your discharge? I would be happy to go over it with you and give you any suggestions that might help."

"Thanks, Doc, that would be great, but I am very worried about Clarence. He's smart; he's a good person, but he is scared shitless. He's got some crazy ideas about knowing something that could get him killed, but I don't think it's so. Nonetheless, he is the one person here that I feel connected with besides you. How can I help you to help him?"

"Let me put my head to work on that. Meanwhile you get working on your own plan and get your thoughts on paper. We'll talk more later about how we together might be able to help Clarence.

Fred got up, looked Wilfred in the eye and said, "Let's get it done." Wilfred smiled back.

Chapter 18:
WANDA AT THE CAFETERIA

Fred sauntered to the cafeteria. Things were generally going well on the ward, and he was feeling positive about his slowly blossoming relationship with Wanda. He looked forward to meeting her for lunch, and to finding out how Marie was doing. He had struck up a warm relationship with Wanda's child, and it was not just to make a connection with her mother. He was genuinely taken by a warm feeling about Marie.

Wanda was already at a table in the cafeteria. When she saw him come in, she waved and pointed to the seat across from her. Fred came over and they both got into the line. Fred put a chicken salad sandwich and a glass of orange juice on his tray. Wanda selected a bowl of chicken soup and a V-8. They put their trays on the table and sat down again. Fred asked how Maria was doing after their recent get-together.

"She was very impressed with you, Fred. She asked when we could have you over for dinner. I think she was trying to play Cupid."

"I was very impressed with her as well, and if that turns into an invitation at some point, you can consider me as having accepted in advance. I enjoy your company, both of you."

"Thanks, Fred, we really liked the evening with you as well. By the way, you did a great job calming things down earlier today. The staff was impressed, and the whole unit relaxed, including the patients. I suspect Dr. Nolan will pick up on it as well, which will be a feather in your cap."

"As far as Nolan goes, I just want to keep out of his way and generally stay invisible. I do have some concerns about a couple of patients on the unit. Jonathon Maxwell is one who will need some vigilance. Hypnosis is a good tool that I can use to work with him – or should I say them. However, Wilfred and Clarence are the ones I need to focus on. Wilfred is close to ready to get out of the hospital and needs some preparation. Clarence is in a stuck place, but he is bright and could make it eventually, if we can get past his delusions.

But, enough about the unit. How are you doing? That was a stressful thing today. You didn't get hurt, did you? And you mentioned a family emergency that kept you off work for a week or so. Is everything OK? Is there anything I can help you with?"

"I'm OK. He was just bluster with the broken chair, but he was getting pretty wound up. You calmed things down nicely.

The family issue had to do with Maria. Her dad and I never married, but he has kept himself in our lives peripherally. He faithfully provides child support but married someone else and now has a couple of kids. Maria knows them and they accept her, but the relationship has always been a little distant. About two weeks ago her dad got some bad medical news. He was diagnosed with leukemia. It hit his family very hard, and it affected us as well, in spite of our rather tangential relationship. Maria really felt badly for his other kids and wanted to be in contact with them. I took some time off to try to be helpful to his wife and kids while he was undergoing tests and treatment. It's not clear what the prognosis is yet. Maria's opportunity to have dinner with you has perked her up quite a bit. It's a complicated situation, but I think she is handling it quite well and starting to connect with her half-siblings in a better way."

Fred was taken aback a little by the mention of the leukemia. His memory shot back about eight years to when his wife was diagnosed. He recalled the pain and fear and the dread associated with it.

"I know how hard that can be on a family, especially one with kids. My wife died of leukemia when I was in medical school. It was a rough spell. Is there a way that I can be helpful to Maria? I would be glad to talk to her about my way of getting through it. A lot of it had to do with feeling very sad but getting the help of family and friends."

"Thanks, Fred. I'll talk to her and maybe we can plan to have you over for dinner one of these evenings. I'll give you a call. I think she would really like that, and so would I.

Well, that was a quick lunch. Time to get back to work. I will definitely call you soon."

They walked quietly but peacefully back to the unit together. When they got to the locked door, Wanda opened it with her key. Fred had the urge to kiss her like he had just taken her home from a date but had to chuckle to himself about how he was feeling.

Chapter 19:
A LETTER FOR CLARENCE

Fred had been working on 2E for almost four months, and Clarence had been there for almost the same amount of time. Things had not changed much for Clarence during that time. He continued to be fearful, kept to himself a great deal, and had a stealthy look about him. There was a wariness about him that resembled a feral cat. On this Tuesday in late August, he seemed particularly rattled. He had received a letter from his parents. It was the first mail that he had received since his arrival. He was afraid to open it. He carried it with him as he paced repeatedly from the dayroom to his room and back. He finally approached Wilfred and asked for his help. Wilfred patiently sat down with him and, using a calm voice, reassured Clarence that he would be there for support while his anxious friend opened the letter and read it. After more hesitation, Clarence opened the letter. As he read it, he became more wide-eyed, and his hands shook visibly. He almost dropped it as he handed it to Wilfred to read.

"Dear son,

We are sorry that we have not written sooner, but we were told, after your experience on the water tower, that it might be best not to contact you until you had become a bit more stable. However, recently we have had someone here who was looking for you. He said that he was a reporter from the New York Times, and we had to tell him that you were in the hospital. He said that he would like to visit you there if he were allowed, so we thought you should be aware of this possibility. Also, not long afterward, we had a visit from two other people who said that they were from the FBI and wanted to speak with you. They too may be in touch. I hope this is nothing serious. We just want you to get well, so talk to the doctors and please follow their advice.

We love you and hope you are getting better.

Mom and Dad

P.S. Mr. Fattorino came by the house to check on how you are doing. He wanted to wish you well."

Wilfred read it and frowned. Clarence was still shaking.

"Clarence, do you have any idea what this is all about? From your reaction, I would guess that you do."

"I think it's related to that mafia thing that I have been worried about. I think it's going to stir up all kinds of trouble for me."

"But how did a reporter from The New York Times get involved? And the FBI?"

"It's probably from that phone call I made when some of us went on the field trip to the museum. Not everyone knows about that. I think only Dr. Quimby knows. I called the Times late at night and they probably talked to the FBI about some of the details I told them. Oh my god, if they start looking for me here to interview me, the mob will find out and come after me here, even if they think I'm crazy! But wait, if Mr. Fattorino knows I am here, they already know anyway. I'm going to have to get out of here sooner than I wanted, but I don't know where I'll go. I can't go home. They'll find me there. I've got to think. I've got to have a plan."

"Calm down, Clarence. Take it easy. You'll be safe here. No one will try to get in here to harm you. The hospital won't let that happen. Dr. Quimby won't let that happen. I will be keeping an eye on you too. You know how I like to keep track of things going on here."

"I've got to let Dr. Quimby know too. He doesn't know anything about this stuff that I know, but the mafia may think he does. They may think that I've been spilling the beans to my doctor all along. They may even try to do something bad to him too. Oh my god, what have I done?"

"You're right Clarence, you should talk with Dr. Quimby about this. He can help you. Just remember that I am in your corner and will help you in any way that I can. Try to keep calm. Remember, panic interferes with your ability to think things through clearly."

"Wilfred, I am afraid to talk to Quimby. I don't want him to get more involved in this than he already is. That letter from my parents ---- right at the end they mention a visit from Mr. Fattorino. He is the man in whose house I did my magic show for his kid's party. He's the one who knows that I have information about his family that could send a lot of people to prison."

"Clarence, I know that letter really set off alarms for you. If you want me to help you, I really need to know more about what happened. You've been holding your cards close to your chest for a long time, but I need to understand enough to give you helpful advice. Please fill me in."

Clarence sighed deeply. "If anyone can help me sort this out, I think you can, professor. You have an uncanny ability to size things up. I've watched you. I can trust you. What I don't want is to put you in danger. I think that you are peripheral enough among my contacts that they would not suspect you to have the kind of information that I am about to tell you.

When I was trying to supplement my income by doing magic, I was hired by the Fattorino family for a surprise birthday party for one of his kids. Because it was a surprise and the kid and his mother were returning late after an afternoon out together, I was ushered into the father's private office to hide until they arrived.

His desktop had several open books, and I couldn't resist looking at them. I didn't fully understand those books, but I knew they were financial in nature. I had this little secret camera that I had bought, and I took a bunch of pictures. It wasn't a good idea, but I was itching to try out my new camera. I heard the door starting to open, so I quickly tucked the camera away and walked away from the desk, but I realized that I had left the books in more disarray than I had found them. I got a funny look from the person who was ushering me to the party room, but we did the party, I got paid, and I was given a ride home.

I was scared. I got the pictures developed within a couple of days and realized they were financial records and they involved lots of money. There was also information about where some of the money was hidden. I went to a bank and opened a safety deposit box in my grandfather's name and put the photos in it. They're still there. Now the journalist from the NY Times and the FBI want to talk to me, and the Fattorino family probably has me in its sights."

"How much did you tell the reporter for the Times over the phone? It must have been just enough for him to try to get more information from the FBI and to do more digging and want to interview you in person."

"I rambled a lot while I was on the phone. I was hiding at the Historical Museum and was trying to get them to put enough in the Times to put pressure on the mob to distract them from me. Eventually, that conversation was interrupted by the police coming to the museum, so I had to cut it off and get out of there. I went to Quimby's home, and he got me back to the hospital. He kind of kept the whole thing pretty much under wraps, I think."

"So how much does the FBI really know and how much do you really know."

"The FBI may have a file on the Fattorinos, but I really don't know for sure. I didn't fully understand the stuff I took pictures of, but I do know where the pictures are, and that may be what they all want.

"I really think you should go over this with Quimby. If you want me to be there when you tell him about it, I am OK with that if he is, but he is the one who can screen who gets to come here and talk to you. Go check in with the nurse and arrange to talk to the doc."

Clarence walked down to the nurses' station. He knocked on the glass and saw that Dr. Quimby was there speaking with the nurses. Clarence said, "Dr. Quimby, we need to talk." Fred said, "Let's go to my office, Clarence."

In the office, showed Fred the letter from his parents and went over his fears about the NY Times, the FBI, and the family he had worked for.

"Doc, I have to get out of this place."

"Clarence, we've been over this before. This fear is exaggerated. Besides these people cannot visit you here without your permission and ours, and we are not about to have reporters and FBI agents in here to disturb our patients. What we really need to do is to help you deal with these fears. Besides, where would you go, what would you do? You would have to have a place to live and a job to support yourself. You would be even more fearful if you left this place right now. Over time, we could help you get set up to be able to take care of yourself. Let's start working on these things."

"But Doc, what if they send an assassin in here to do the job?"

"That's a bit over the top, don't you think, Clarence?"

"It's not unheard of, Doc. Somebody could act crazy and get admitted."

"Isn't that a bit far-fetched, Clarence?"

"I got into this place that way, Doc. It's not that far-fetched."

"All right, Clarence. Let's start by limiting your visitors. Clearly, we'll have no reporters or FBI agents. Do you want your parents to be able to come here to see you? Let's leave it strictly to just your parents then. I will instruct the nurses to give you a mild sedative in the meantime to help you calm down, Okay?"

"Okay, Doc, let's leave it at that for now. Thanks."

Clarence left Fred's office and headed for the dayroom.

Fred went to the nurses' station to order some meds for Clarence.

Chapter 20:
TWO WEEKS LATER

Quimby walked onto the ward on Monday morning feeling generally well about his time on 2E. He had about two months left on the unit before transferring down to the University hospital across town to finish his first year of residency. He had successfully helped to negotiate a discharge for Wilfred Donne with Dr. Nolan. He was making good progress with Jonathon Maxwell and his troupe. Clarence had a visit with his parents about a week ago and was making progress and looking in much better spirits. When Fred walked into the nurses' station, he was met by Wanda who had a perplexed look on her face.

"Dr. Quimby, we had a bit of a surprise over the weekend. Clarence Jensen managed to elope from the hospital some time Saturday night and has not been found. I know you would have wanted to know, even on the weekend, but I did not find out until I arrived on the unit for this morning's shift."

"Wow! Does anyone know how it happened? He seemed to be doing so well since he had contact with his family."

"Apparently one of the new orderlies is missing his key to the unit and Clarence was just gone on Sunday morning."

"Clarence has proven to be quite adept at picking pockets. He has gotten my keys a couple of times in a joking fashion but has always returned them to me immediately. Did he leave any kind of message?"

While Wanda and Fred were talking, Rudy walked up to Fred and handed him a note.

"Clarence told me to give this to you when you came in this morning, Dr. Q."

Fred unfolded the paper and read, "Dr. Q., I have decided after speaking with my parents that the best course for me is to leave the hospital and change my identity. I'll find a job and place to stay on my own. I will probably be in touch with you sometime, but I am not sure exactly when. I hope you stay safe. I think for your sake that it is best that I leave and not risk placing you in any more danger. Thanks for your help and friendship. You know that I am capable of reaching you. I found you before."

Fred showed it to Wanda.

"Do you think you should show this to Dr. Nolan?"

"I think I had better keep it to myself. Nolan may blow a gasket if he associates me with this."

After Fred let the news about Clarence sink in, Wanda said,

"Well, Fred, on a different subject, Maria and I wondered if you could join us for dinner next Saturday evening? She's been really wanting to talk to you about leukemia, and I just want you over for your company. I think the leukemia thing is just a starter for her. She really wants your company as well."

"That sounds great. Should I bring some wine? And – what does Maria like for a beverage?"

"Just bring yourself. I'll supply the wine and chocolate milk for Maria. Is six o'clock Okay?"

"Sounds fine, but I'll need the address."

Wanda wrote her address down on a small note paper and handed it to Fred.

"Thanks, I'll be looking forward to a nice evening."

Fred went about his Monday rounds musing about Clarence and what he would be up to next, but smiling to himself about the upcoming weekend with Wanda and Maria.

Chapter 21:
DINNER WITH THE LADIES

Fred showed up a little early at the small house near the University. It even had a picket fence around the front. He brought a book for Maria, that he hoped she was old enough to appreciate, Madeleine L'Engle's children's novel, *A Wrinkle in Time*. Two fresh cut long-stem roses were also included for the hostess. He tried not to overdress and wore a dress shirt and slacks but did not spare the cologne. He rang the bell, and the door immediately was opened by Maria.

"Hello Fred", Maria beamed. "Ooo, flowers!"

"And how is my favorite six-year-old?"

"I'm fine. We're both excited to have you for dinner tonight. We had such a good time last time."

Maria whispered, "Mom worked especially hard to make a nice lasagna dinner. I hope you like Italian food."

"Your mom must be a good detective. I love Italian food. By the way, I brought you something I hope you'll like." He handed her the book.

"Oooh, I've heard about this book. Thank you. I've just started *The Lion, The Witch and The Wardrobe* by C.S. Lewis, and I'll get right into this one as soon as I finish it."

Wanda's voice from within the house called, "Maria, please bring Fred in so I can talk to him too. Things are all set up to relax and have a little time before the lasagna is ready."

Fred and Maria joined Wanda in their small living room off the kitchen. Wanda opened a bottle of Cabernet for her and Fred and poured a ginger-ale for Maria. Fred commented about her detective work regarding the Italian dinner, and she giggled a little and said that

Dr. Nolan had let something slip about Fred's Italian heritage, so she took a chance.

The evening went well, the food was excellent, and around 8 o'clock, it was time for Maria to go to bed. She was disappointed and somewhat reluctant to end her part of the evening, but asked Wanda if Fred could tuck her in while mom cleaned up the dishes from dinner. Fred smiled and looked at Wanda who smiled back and nodded. "You go get your jammies on and then come out and get Fred." Maria ran off to her bedroom and was back in a moment in her pajamas.

As Fred tucked Maria into bed, she looked at him and said, "I like you a lot, Fred. Do you like my mommy? I hope so. I don't know my daddy very well, and he is very sick, but I wish you like mommy a lot and maybe could be a daddy for me."

Fred was taken a little bit by surprise. He said, "I like you a lot too, Maria, and I like your mommy, but you know when people make those kinds of decisions about being together, both people have to decide that and want it to happen."

Maria grinned and said, "I can tell from watching mommy that she likes you, and I bet she would like for you to be my other daddy."

Fred leaned over and gave Maria a little kiss on the forehead and said, "That would be nice, but we will have to see if things will fall into place like that. No matter what, we will always be friends, and that is a pinky promise." Fred reached his little finger out to hook up with hers. "Have sweet dreams." She smiled up at him and closed her eyes. He watched her for a moment as she drifted off.

Fred joined Wanda in the living room.

"You've got quite the girl in there. She is bright for her age and very astute. I wondered if the book I brought her would be a little too old for her, but I knew you could read it to her; then she told me she was reading a C.S. Lewis book."

"Yes, she keeps me on my toes, and in spite of the myriad of feelings she sometimes shows about her father's health, she keeps her spirits up fairly well."

"How is her dad doing? Have you heard anything about his treatment? Do they let you in on that?

"From what I can gather, things are pretty grim. There is some talk about doing a bone marrow transplant, but the difficulty is finding a match from a donor. So far, they have not had much luck."

"How many have they tried?"

"About four or five so far, I think, but his white counts are starting to drop and that's not a good sign."

"If they are OK with it, I could get tested to see if I am a match."

"That's very kind, Fred. I can check with them to see."

"Anything to help you and Maria, and obviously the guy who needs it the most. It's not a very extensive procedure, I understand. Please do check on it."

Fred watched Wanda's somber expression and changed the subject.

"Now on a different subject, that was a fabulous dinner tonight, and I thoroughly enjoyed the evening with you two. I didn't get to talk to Maria much about her father or the leukemia, but she was quite clear, in a more than direct way, that she wanted me to be around in her life. I must say that I was both surprised and thrilled."

"What did she say?" Wanda looked a bit flushed.

"Maria said she liked me a lot and hoped that I liked her mommy a lot, so that maybe I could be a daddy for her. I told her that was a decision that grown-up people would have to make. I did make her another pinky promise that no matter what is decided, she and I will always be friends."

Wanda flushed visibly. "Fred, I did not put her up to this. I am embarrassed that we started this friendship in such a weird way. I do like you a lot, and I don't want you to think that I am putting thoughts in her head."

"Not to worry. I am grateful and thankful for you letting me into both of your lives. I would do anything I can to help you both."

Fred reached out, pulled her to him and kissed her. She relaxed and savored his kiss.

"Now I would like to help you clean up so we can do the dishes."

Fred got home considerably later than he had expected he would that night.

Chapter 22:
A SURPRISE CONTACT

The following Monday Fred had called the unit to tell them that he would be late. He had to make a stop at Mercy Hospital in town before coming to work to check on something there. He was up late reading the night before, so he slept in as long as he dared and stopped at his usual coffee stand to get an espresso to bump his energy level. While standing behind a customer waiting for his coffee, he heard a voice behind him saying,

"Can you spare a buck for a coffee and donut, mister? I haven't had a decent meal for a few days and am totally broke."

The voice sounded familiar. He turned and did not at first recognize the man in the rumpled fedora with long blond hair. The man looked gaunt and hungry, so Fred reached for his wallet to extract a dollar to give to the man, but his wallet was missing. He quickly checked his other pockets and began to look around as though he may have dropped it.

"Is this what you are looking for?" The stranger handed him the wallet.

"Oh, thank goodness. Where did you find it?"

There was just a cryptic smile on the stranger's face, which now began to look surprisingly familiar.

Fred took the wallet and pulled out a five-dollar bill and handed it to the man in gratitude.

"Thanks, Doc." was the reply. It was Clarence.

"Clarence, what are you up to? Picking my pocket again, you scoundrel? That's a hell of a way to reintroduce yourself. Are you OK? Where are you staying? Do your parents know you are safe? What are your plans?" How have you been since you left the hospital? No more worries about being poisoned?"

"Whoa, Doc, one at a time. I am hoping to find a way to make some money. I would like to get a job. If I could find Wilfred, he may be able to help me find a place to stay. Do you have any idea where I could locate him? It's been kind of exciting out here in the streets. I'm not worried, because I am now anonymous, but I do miss Wilfred. I was a bit surprised to run into you in this neighborhood."

Fred hesitated, but he knew that the two were friends, so he told Clarence that Wilfred had landed a job at the library where his knowledge of books made him somewhat of an expert. Clarence could try to locate him there.

Fred knew that Clarence knew where he lived, but he was not about to invite him to his apartment, even though he felt sorry for him. That could be a disaster if someone discovered that he was harboring an escapee from the hospital who was also his patient. Then he thought of Maria's father and suggested that Clarence might consider looking into donating bone marrow or plasma for some short-term cash. Fred slipped an extra $5 to Clarence and suggested he could follow Fred to Mercy Hospital if he was interested in donating tissue. "I am on my way there right now to check on the same thing. I know someone who needs a bone marrow transplant."

Clarence thought donating tissue or blood for short-term cash sounded like a decent plan. Together they walked the block and a half to the hospital. At the main desk, they inquired where the hematology department was located. On the fourth floor they inquired about donating. Fred had checked with Wanda about the name of Maria's father so he could specifically ask about donating to him if he were a match. He decided to include Clarence in that match attempt as well. Maria's father's name was Ronald Torkensen. The nurse was happy to take blood samples from both Fred and Clarence, who was now using the name, Karl Johnson. She said she would not have the results back for a couple of days. They would have to come back then, and if they matched a need, more tests would be done for a marrow transplant. Blood could also be donated at that time, depending on type and absence of any pathology.

They left the hematology department together. Fred asked Clarence what he was up to next.

"I think I am going to try to see if I can locate Wilfred at the library to see if he might be able to put me up for a while until I get a job. I'll check back here in a couple of days to follow up. Thanks, Doc, for the financial infusion and the information." He abruptly turned a corner, walked briskly, turned another corner and was gone.

Fred pondered the whole encounter and continued to be amazed at how well Clarence had disguised himself and now seemed much more confident in his ability to survive with his new-found "anonymity". Leaving the so-called security that he had imagined in the hospital had done more to improve his outlook and diminish his fear than several months on the unit.

Chapter 23:
REUNION

Clarence found a phone book in a drug store and looked up the address of the public library. It was only a few blocks away, and he got there in a manner of minutes. At the main desk he said that he had to deliver a message to Wilfred Donne. She had him wait while she sent someone to the stacks to find Wilfred. Five minutes later, Wilfred appeared, looking energized and fresh. He looked quizzically at Clarence until his visitor spoke.

"Well, professor, I entered the ocean, and you were right, I became part of it and lost my fear."

"You read the poem. I am so glad it helped. What are you up to? Where are you staying?"

"I hope to find a job so I can afford a place to stay. I ran into Doc Quimby who told me where to find you. I hope that's OK. He knew we were friends at the hospital. He gave me a few bucks to get by for a little while. I must tell you that my newfound anonymity has freed me up."

Wilfred grinned. "Clarence, you can stay with me. I have a one-bedroom apartment, but I also have a hide-a-bed couch. I have some extra clothes that could fit you, and we could clean you up a bit. We could manage together for a while until you get on your feet. It would be good company. My manager here at the library was just talking about needing to hire someone to help in the stacks, so there might even be a job for you here. The pay isn't all that great, but you wouldn't need much for starters."

"I don't want to put you out, but I like the idea of hanging out with you till I get on my feet. I went to the hospital with Doc to get set up to donate blood or bone marrow for a little money if I need it. I'll go back there in a couple of days to see how the screening tests turned out."

Wilfred told Clarence he would be off work at five. Clarence said he had enough money to get some lunch. He said he would like to check out the library, do some reading, and later they could go together to Wilfred's place. Wilfred nodded approval and proposed that they pick up some KFC on the way home.

Chapter 24:
HEMATOLOGY LAB

The weather was getting a bit nippy as the season was getting close to Thanksgiving. Clarence was glad that Wilfred had some extra wool shirts and a jacket he could borrow. The last couple of days were the most comfortable he had experienced in some time. Wilfred was an easy host. Clarence did his best to make his stay easy on his friend by helping out wherever he could. They talked about books, the library, and what was in the newspaper, but rarely about their time in the hospital. Wilfred was doing some lobbying for Clarence about a job at the library, but today Clarence was on his way to the hospital to check on the lab tests in hopes that he might come up with a little cash by donating blood or marrow.

He checked in at the hematology desk and took a seat. A lab tech called his name, brought him to a room with file drawers of records and pulled one out.

"Karl Johnson?" Clarence nodded.

"Very interesting, Mr. Johnson, you are a perfect match for a bone marrow transplant for Mr. Torkensen. We have been trying to find a match for him for a while now, and he really needs one."

"What kind of a procedure is it?"

"Well, it's fairly simple. We either make a small cut into your hip or your sternum and take out some marrow from the bone. It is a clean surgical procedure and not too uncomfortable. Most people do it from the bone just above the hip."

"And what kind of pay is there for this procedure?"

"Well, usually it is a donation."

"But the Red Cross pays for blood donations all the time. This sounds a bit more complicated than a needle in the arm."

"Well, I would have to speak with my supervisor. Our patient is in dire need of a transplant. Dr. Peterson may be willing to speak with you about your request."

Dr. Peterson was aware that time was short for Mr. Torkensen without a bone marrow transplant. He agreed to pay this Mr. Johnson one hundred and twenty dollars if he was willing to donate today. He did not want to lose this valuable donor. Clarence haggled with him until the agreed upon amount was one hundred and fifty dollars. Clarence wanted enough money to help Wilfred put together a nice Thanksgiving meal for the two of them.

The procedure was arranged within the hour. Both Clarence and Dr. Peterson were pleased with the arrangement, and by late afternoon Clarence was walking back to Wilfred's place, his hip a little tender but with the money in his pocket.

Late that afternoon, Fred Quimby called the hematology department at the hospital to find out if he was a match for the marrow transplant. He was disappointed to find out that he was not. They did not tell him about their good luck with finding another donor.

Chapter 25:
WINDING DOWN ON UNIT 2E

Back on the unit with Thanksgiving around the corner, Fred was trying to get his patients to a point where they could be discharged or where their care could be summarized for the next resident to take over in January. As he sat in the nursing station going over charts, Wanda came in. Fred looked up and saw that she seemed in good spirits and said, "I went to hematology at Mercy Hospital and got tested for the bone marrow transplant, but I was not a match."

She looked at him and smiled. "I just got a call from the other family last evening and was told that they did find someone who was a match, and they arranged for the transplant to take place last evening. Apparently, it was a person who was indigent and looking to sell his blood. It just happened that he was a perfect marrow match for Ron. They jumped on the opportunity and got Ron in ASAP."

Fred didn't mention Clarence, but he couldn't help but wonder if he was the donor. "Wow, that is marvelous. I sure hope it works out. You must be excited. Does Maria know?"

"Not yet. We didn't want to get her excited until we saw whether the treatment worked or not, but I am hopeful for her. She hadn't been really close with the family until her father got ill, but she has made some very empathic connections with his other kids since then."

"You know, when the residents rotate in January, I will be downtown at the main University psychiatric unit, and we won't have to be so careful about Dr. Nolan's rules about relationships among staff. Meanwhile, I would like to celebrate Thanksgiving with you and Maria. Would you like to go out to a nice dinner later in the afternoon at a special restaurant – my treat?"

"We would really like that, provided you come back to our place afterwards for a nice dessert, and maybe a nice bottle of wine – my treat.

Maria will be very excited. She was asking me if we could have you over again sometime soon."

"Sounds like a plan. I will make reservations at a nice place. When I get the details, I'll let you know. I'll look forward to a nice day with you both. Meanwhile, I had better get busy and put some finishing touches on some of my work on the unit before I make the transition to downtown. Back to the salt mine."

Fred grabbed a few charts and sauntered down to his office.

One of the cases that still needed work was that of Jonathon Maxwell, the man with the multiple personality disorder. Things had gone reasonably smoothly for a while, but in addition to Peter, the child, Jack the teenager, Randolph the "manager", and Jonathon, whose personality still did not seem to have a clue about some of the others, several additional personalities had slipped out.

Fred's main approach would be to maintain a strong helpful relationship with Randolph, who seemed to be most aware of all the other personalities. Then he would have to find ways to bring the other personalities into awareness of each other. He hoped to get them to cooperate to make their interactions with one another more productive and less likely to get them all in trouble.

Fred's way of approaching this was to remind each one that they "all lived in the same house" and if one of them got evicted by going to jail, they all suffered the consequences. This was particularly pointed out if one of the personalities ended up in an isolation room after acting out. Fred would wait for the alter to cool down, go into the room, sit quietly, and begin to look at alternative choices that could have been made with a better outcome. Sometimes it worked and sometimes it didn't seem to have much impact, depending on the alter and the issue.

Fred had become reasonably good at using hypnosis as a tool with some of the personalities, but he knew that it would be particularly important to have a face-to-face conference with whoever took his place on the unit, about this particular patient, rather than just leaving notes in his chart. He made it a point to make that offer in the chart notes.

Fred kept thinking about Clarence. He wondered if Clarence was the marrow match for Maria's father, and if he ever connected with Wilfred. Fred couldn't help but be concerned for him. He did feel better about what appeared to be Clarence's new sense of release from some of his fears, but he also tended to see Clarence as potentially fragile.

Fred tried to focus on the charts, but he kept getting distracted by thinking about Clarence and Wilfred, and by the realization that he was falling in love with Wanda, and the thought of having a family with her and Maria. He finally packed up the charts, brought them back to the nursing station, and left early to go downtown to his seminars.

Chapter 26:
THANKSGIVING PREPARATIONS

Fred looked for a comfortable restaurant that would serve tasty meals that would appeal both to Wanda and to a young girl. He found a good Italian place that would be perfect and made a reservation for three at five o'clock on Thanksgiving Day. They not only served the usual pasta dishes and Italian sausage, but also served specialty dishes of fish, lamb, veal, and vegetarian. He wanted to make it just right. He also visited jewelry stores, searching for a nice small gift for Wanda. As he sauntered about with his head in the clouds, he heard a familiar voice.

"Can you spare a buck for a coffee and a donut, Mister?"

Clarence had a knack for sudden surprises.

"Clarence, what brings you to this end of town?"

"Oh, I'm just running some errands for Wilfred. He is tied up with his job at the library, so I picked up his laundry and now I'm on my way to get some groceries for our Thanksgiving dinner. I was just joking about the coffee and donut. I was able to get some money at the blood bank. It turned out that I was a match for a particular bone marrow they were looking for. Wilfred was also able to pull some strings at the library to get me a job there. It's minimum wage, but enough to get me by for the time being, especially since he is also letting me room with him until I am on my feet."

"I am glad to hear that. I think I know of the person who needed the marrow donation. He is an acquaintance of one of the nurses on the unit. Sounds like they were very grateful for what could be a life-saving gift. Are you still feeling comfortable being out and about with your anonymity?"

"As long as I am not spending a lot of time in the public eye, I am OK. I work in the stacks at the library with Wilfred. If I were employed somewhere that had a lot of foot traffic in a public place, I might be a bit more anxious."

"I am spending some time with a woman who has a young daughter. If I ever needed you for a magic party for her to celebrate something special, would you be willing to help me out? I am sure you still have it in you."

"You know me, Doc, if it pays enough and is not a big splashy party with Italian big shots, I would help out."

"So is the library the best place to reach you?"

"Yes, for now. Just ask for Wilfred, and he will know how to find me or get a message to me. Tell Wanda that I hope the marrow works for her friend. I assume it is Wanda. I didn't know that she had a daughter."

"Nothing slips by you, does it, Clarence?

"Well, she's the prettiest nurse on the unit, and you have always had a bit of a deference towards her. It only makes sense. Of all the nurses on the unit, she is also the kindest."

"Clarence, starting in January I will be transferred to the University Hospital. Most of my time will be on the inpatient unit there, but I will also be given a few hours a week to do some outpatient work. If you ever need someone to talk to about any issues, I could probably be available to see you there. I just say this to give you some options if you need them. Anyway, it was good to see you again. I have to scoot now, but good luck, and I hope we'll run into one another from time to time."

"Adios for now, Doc, and thanks for the offer. I might well take you up on it. You may see me sooner than you think."

Chapter 27:
THANKSGIVING

Fred drove to Wanda and Maria's home about 4:15 on Thanksgiving Day with a bouquet of 6 red roses. Wanda was smartly but casually dressed. Maria had a new fall coat on and looked pleased to see him. Fred wore a sport jacket but over a turtleneck.

They drove to Luigi's restaurant, parked the car, and got there a few minutes early for the reservation. At their table, Fred could not help but pick up on a strong sense of anticipation in Maria. She scanned the menu but put it down quickly and said, "I want to have some ravioli."

Wanda looked at her and asked, "Would you like some salad before the ravioli? They have some great looking salads, too."

Maria said, "I do like salad, but I'm afraid I might fill up on the salad and not have room for the ravioli."

Fred popped in and said, "It's OK, Maria, whatever you don't finish, you can have them box it up and take it home for the next day. Order whatever looks good. Then you can be thankful two days in a row."

The dinner went well. Maria enjoyed about half of her ravioli after devouring most of her salad. Wanda had a nice Walleye pike, and Fred enjoyed spaghetti with Italian sausage. The conversation was spirited, and yet, throughout the dinner, Fred was aware of a sense of anticipation in Maria. When they had finished, the waiter boxed up the rest of Maria's ravioli, and Fred paid the check and got their coats. Wanda reminded Fred that she had picked up a nice bottle of wine to go with dessert at home, and they were on their way.

At home, Wanda put on some music, got some wine glasses, and opened a nice bottle of Pinot Noir, imported all the way from Oregon. She said she had done some research on wines before buying it by asking a good friend who is into fine wines. Her friend also told her where she could get some pre-made Panna Cotta dessert, and when Wanda brought it to the table, it looked scrumptious.

Maria was smiling, but quiet. Fred looked at her and said, "Maria, did all that ravioli make you tired or sleepy?"

"No, I'm sorry for not being more happy. I am just worried about my father. He has been very sick and it is hard to be super thankful on Thanksgiving when I don't know if he will get better."

"From what I understand, the kind of illness he has is being studied very hard and they are learning some new ways of treating it, so it is possible that he might come out of this sickness."

Wanda entered into the conversation. "I didn't tell you this earlier, because we don't know yet what the results will be, but your dad did get a special treatment a few days ago that might have a chance of getting him better. We just have to give it some time to find out. A man donated a part of his own blood making tissue to put into your dad to see if it would fix him. Fred also tried to do that, but it wasn't the right type for dad."

"Wow, you tried to do that for my dad? Thank you!"

"OK, let's not get ahead of ourselves here. There are a lot of people working hard to try to help your dad. Let's just put our worries aside for a while and let the helpers do their work of helping. And I don't know about you two, but my mouth is watering just thinking about those fancy desserts that your mom got for us. How about we dig into those Panna Cotta."

After eating the desserts, Maria looked beat. It was an emotional day for her, both with excitement about going out to dinner and worrying about her dad. Wanda told her to get into her pajamas and then come to say goodnight. Wanda relaxed and thanked Fred for how he had handled Maria's concerns.

Fred looked at her and said, "You know, I ran into Clarence again today and as it turned out, he was the donor match for Maria's father. I had run into him on my way to try to be a donor myself. He was looking for a way to make some money, so he joined me and got tested. He told me today that he was a positive match for the man for whom they were looking. Talk about a small world."

"Wow, that is amazing! Our Clarence who eloped from the hospital? What a circle of life that is. We are so blessed to have you in our lives, Fred, not just for the wonderful luck that you bring, but for your friendship and caring."

"Well, keep that thought, Wanda, because I picked up a little gift for you today." Fred took a small package out of his pocket and told her to open it. Inside was a modest ring. He said, "We had an inauspicious beginning, but I have had the good fortune of falling in love with you and with your daughter. I would like very much to spend my life with you. Would you please marry me?"

"Before I answer you, I need to do something."

She got up, went into Maria's room, and brought out a sleepy-eyed girl.

"Maria, Fred just asked me if I would marry him. I wanted to answer him with you here too. Yes, Fred, I would be honored to marry you. I do love you, and I know Maria would also be happy to have you be in our lives as a family."

Maria walked over to Fred and gave him a big hug. "That makes me very happy, Fred. Can I call you Daddy Fred?"

"Sure Maria, but we had better wait until it is official before you start calling me that. But for now, you are looking very sleepy. Can I tuck you in to your bed?"

"Yes, but I don't want to wake up in the morning thinking this was all just a dream."

"Well, I'll tell you what. I am going to take one of these red roses out of the bouquet of flowers that I brought when I came to pick you up tonight, and I am going to put it on your nightstand so you will remember that everything that happened here tonight was for real and not a dream, OK?"

"Yes, and when I wake up in the morning, I am going to ask Mom how I can freeze it so it will keep forever --right Mom?"

Wanda smiled.

Fred walked Maria back to her room, tucked her in and gave her a kiss on her forehead. She looked at him and said, "Thanks for a special evening, Daddy Fred." And closed her eyes.

When he returned to Wanda, she looked at him and said, "I would like to toast our engagement with this nice bottle of wine that I found, and I would like you to spend the night." Fred grinned.

Chapter 28:
NEW ROTATION
January 1970

Fred's new placement officially started on New Years Day, but he was scheduled to report for orientation on Friday, the following day. He was relieved that he did not catch on call duties on the first weekend. He would be able to review charts to see what he would be facing on the first Monday on the new assignment. He was to report to a senior resident, who essentially ran the details of the ward under the eye of the attending psychiatrist. His duties would be much like what they had been on 2E at the state hospital, but the patient population tended to be more acute with shorter stays. In addition, he would have one afternoon a week when he would be assigned to outpatient responsibilities. Most of these patients would be recently discharged, but sometimes involved individuals who had little or no insurance and who needed care.

It had been a bit of a whirlwind finishing up on 2E. Nevertheless, he had managed to make time to consult with his replacement about Jonathon Maxwell and his alter personalities, and to offer his own observations and suggestions to the new resident. Christmas had gone well with Wanda and Maria, and fortunately the marrow transplant with Maria's father had also gone well, and he seemed to be in remission – at least so far.

It was Fred's third day in his new job. His afternoon for seeing outpatients fell on Wednesdays, and today was his baptism of fire. He looked at his schedule and saw that he had only three patients on the list at 1:15, 2:30 and 3:45. The first two were people who had been discharged from his new unit two weeks before he got there, and the last was someone named Karl Johnson. That last name rang a bell, but he couldn't place it.

The first two patients were rather routine – checking medications, looking for side effects, making sure support systems were in place, and evaluating mood stability. He checked about any other needs and determined whether to schedule further follow-up here or elsewhere.

When the last patient of the afternoon was due, Fred noticed that there was no paperwork showing a previous admission or previous outpatient care. This surprised him a bit. When the patient entered the room, Fred thought he looked familiar, but he had a beard and mustache and what looked like a toupee.

"Hi doc. Good to see you again." It was Clarence.

"Well Clarence, you're getting better and better at your disguises. How are you getting along? How was your Thanksgiving and Christmas? Are you still rooming with Wilfred? Tell me a little about your world and then tell me how I can help you."

"Wilfred, or as I like to call him, 'The Professor', and I had a very nice Thanksgiving. I was able to help with the cost of the food, thanks to the blood clinic. Neither one of us focus a lot on celebrating Christmas, except to have a nice meal like we did on Thanksgiving, but I did get him a new hat and he gave me a new pair of gloves. My job at the library doesn't pay a lot, but Wilfred lets me room with him for helping with the cooking and cleaning and chipping in whatever I can afford toward expenses. He is a good roommate, and I have learned a lot from him.

The Professor is a very good teacher as well. I learn a lot from him without feeling as though he is going out of his way to instruct me. I guess that's the best way to learn. He sort of sneaks up on you.

I used to be afraid of getting out in the world, but Wilfred said that I was like a river meandering down the mountains and through the meadows. I was afraid to enter the ocean for fear that I would be swallowed up, but I've learned that instead, I've just become a part of something bigger. I'm not so afraid anymore. I'm trying to sort out for myself what kind of a job or career to pursue. I've learned more about myself since I left the hospital and my friendship with the professor has deepened.

I've always been good at sleight of hand things, but short of a career as a pickpocket, which would likely be short-lived, or a magician, which would probably be a dead-end job, there is not much to do with magic, short of entertaining friends. I have also learned that I have what the Professor calls an eidetic memory. Things that I see or hear just stick in my head, and that could possibly come in handy in some careers."

"You're also pretty good at disguises" offered Fred, "and that might come in handy if you were working for a private investigator." Fred let that sink in and then said, "Tell me what made you decide to make an appointment to come in to see me at the clinic. Are you having any concerns that I can help with? Are you still afraid of the mafia or someone trying to do you harm?"

"That's pretty much on the back burner. Since I left the hospital and joined the real world, I have a better sense of anonymity and am comfortable being myself, even when I'm not in disguise. I am grateful to the professor for giving me another perspective on that. I'm also grateful to you, Doc, but what I really need from you now, is the opportunity to have someone to connect with on a regular basis for a while, and maybe periodically after that. – just to keep me on track and recharge my batteries when they need it. That way I won't make myself into a pain in the ass to the professor, and we can just be friends and he doesn't have to be my counselor. Is that something we can agree to do?"

"I think that is a good plan, Clarence. By the way, you should know that the person to whom you donated your bone marrow has had some early success with his illness as a result. My friend who knows the person who needed the transplant told me he is in remission so far."

"Your friend nurse Wanda on 2E, right? I have eyes, Doc. I saw you warming up to her from early in your time on the unit. As time went by the temperature went up.

It's Okay. I didn't mention it to anyone, except maybe the professor, so you won't get in any trouble for fraternizing with the staff. Besides, why else would you be so eager to donate your bone marrow unless you had a special connection to someone who needed it? You weren't doing it for the money like I was."

"Maybe a job working for a private investigator would be right up your alley, Clarence. Have you re-connected with your parents since leaving the hospital?"

"I called them once about two weeks after I left the hospital to see if people were still looking to talk to me, and also to reassure them that I was OK and not doing anything crazy. Mr. Fattorino had called again, but they told him that I had left the hospital and moved out of town. He didn't push it. He is still on my mind, but I have safely put away any evidence that I have in a safe place, and it is a kind of insurance for me. I'm not really obsessing about it like I was, and, like you said, I am pretty good at changing my appearance."

Clarence and Fred caught up for the next thirty minutes or so, and Fred could see that the level of anxiety in Clarence had lowered considerably. He thought the plan to keep in touch and to be professionally available to Clarence was a good move. He also thought to himself that at some point it might prove useful to have Clarence make a connection with the man he had helped with the transplant. The more Fred thought about it, he began to muse about what Maria's father did for a living. He hadn't wanted to ask and nose into Wanda's past life too much, but now he was curious, given Clarence's involvement.

Before he left, Clarence looked at Fred and asked, "Dr. Q, what can you tell me about stuff like LSD and peyote and magic mushrooms? They seem to be the rage among younger people these days, and I was hoping that you could give me some realistic information about these so-called psychedelics."

"You need to be careful around that stuff, Clarence, especially LSD. It's quite potent in small amounts and people can have what are called 'bad trips' and sometimes become psychotic, with hallucinations and distortions of reality. Peyote and magic mushrooms have been used in various native religious ceremonies. They also tend to distort experiences and to give a false sense of time. Various other senses like color and hearing can also be affected. Not something to play around with, especially after having some of the anxieties that you've been dealing with."

"Ever tried them, Doc?"

"No, Clarence, they're illegal, and I don't want to risk my career. I've heard too many stories about people who didn't fully come back from their experiences."

"Like going to hell and not coming back, huh Doc? Weren't you ever curious? I imagine some people would have enough of a sense of adventure that they might want to take the risk."

"My advice would be to steer clear of that stuff, Clarence. Meanwhile we should reschedule. Shall we aim for next week?"

"Sounds good to me, Doc. See you then."

Chapter 29:
A WEEK LATER

Clarence was back for another visit under his newly assumed alias of Karl Johnson. He was excited and seemed to be anticipating something that he wanted to talk about. Fred listened as Clarence began to talk excitedly.

"Remember when we talked last week about psychedelics? Well, I sat down with Wilfred after dinner that night, and we had a long conversation about them. It turns out that he had tried some of them when he was having a bad time in his marriage. Given his state of mind at the time, it didn't sit well with him. However, he told me that he had known some people who had taken them when they were feeling much more positive and had what he called a revelatory experience. It really made me curious, and I wondered if something like that kind of experience might not help me to experience myself in a more energetic and positive way, instead of the 'slinking in the shadows' kind of person I have been. Taking a chance on an adventure like that might even help me to grow my spirit and expand my horizons."

"Last week you brought up the possibility that the experience might be like 'going to hell and not coming back', Clarence. People don't know how they are going to respond to these substances until after they try them. So, it's probably not a good idea to mess around with this stuff when you have struggled with the fears you have had, especially just as you are now starting to get past them."

"Or maybe it's just what I need, Doc. Chasing my demons to hell and leaving them there. I need to be doing something with my life to get out of the shadows."

"Don't look for the magic way out, Clarence. You of all people would know the illusions of magic and how unreal they really are."

"But if you don't try it, you'll never really know, will you Doc?"

"Okay, but if you play Russian Roulette, you won't really know whether or not the bullet is in the chamber until it's too late, will you Clarence?"

"Damn it, Doc. You do have a rather graphic way of putting things in perspective, don't you?"

"So, other than the thought of using something artificial to get your courage up, have you given any thought to where your plans for some kind of a career or job direction might go?"

"I really don't know quite where to start, Doc. I have spoken to the professor about it. His main interests have always been in literature and in teaching, but that's nowhere up my alley. I like doing things and investigating how things are made or done, but I just have a high school education."

"But you do have skills. You do have a good memory. You are perceptive and curious. Are you good with your hands? Have you ever thought about going to a career counselor? Someone who knows about different careers and what it takes to do well in them? Someone like that might have a smorgasbord of things that could be appealing and might be a good fit for you. I could help you to get to someone like that."

"Couldn't you do that for me, Doc? I don't want to start with someone new, and you know my background. Besides, you have already given me some good ideas about maybe working with a private investigator. That sounds intriguing."

"I don't really have the resources at my fingertips that a career counselor would have and would know about. I can help you with some ideas, but it wouldn't be as comprehensive. It is really up to you, Clarence."

"Let's just leave it in your hands for now, OK Doc?"

They talked awhile longer about his family, upbringing, friends, school, and intimacy in his life. His parents had immigrated from Norway right after World War II. Apparently, the grandfather had been in some kind of trouble because of his position with the Nazi occupiers, and the rest of the family had difficulty there until his father arranged for them to get out of the country via Sweden. Clarence was quite young when they came to the U.S., and his family always seemed to be reticent to socialize a lot and tended to keep to themselves. There was an undercurrent in the family of avoiding attention and keeping under the radar. Clarence, for the most part, tended to maintain that surreptitious quality, but on occasion, his need for adventure would herniate out, but then be pushed back in place out of fear.

This one-on-one contact time with Clarence allowed Fred to better understand how Clarence's background and family culture affected his approach to life in general. Fred was getting to know him much better, and Clarence was becoming more comfortable and trusting. They decided to continue with weekly visits for a while.

Chapter 30:
THERAPY HIATUS
February 25

After a couple of more weeks of meetings, it became obvious to both Fred and Clarence that there was no need to continue to meet weekly. Clarence was scratching for things to talk about, and they would be caught up on events in about ten minutes of the session. If Fred tried to dig too deeply into family issues, Clarence was still wary and tended to avoid or change the subject. Fred suggested they meet about once a month; Clarence thought maybe every two weeks. They settled on every three weeks with use of a phone call or adding in more sessions if there were issues that came up needing more immediate attention. Clarence found that he could depend on Wilfred's wisdom to sort out his thoughts on a day-to-day basis. He didn't think he'd need to call Fred.

Clarence was still fascinated by the thought of delving into mind altering substances. He was also caught up in the climate of student protests against the Viet Nam war. On campus, various organizations like Students for a Democratic Society and the Student Nonviolent Coordinating Committee were frequently in the news. As he and Wilfred were watching the evening news, the situation at Cal State Fullerton came on. About twenty police officers came to break up about three hundred war protestors, and all hell broke loose. Anti-war protests were growing across the country, and Clarence looked at the professor and said, "What are your thoughts about this war?"

"I was in the army when the Korean war broke out, and we were sent over there. It was different. The North Koreans invaded the south, who were our allies. In Viet Nam, we invaded them. Maybe we should have left well enough alone. A lot of people have been drafted to fight a war that they probably don't feel the need to be involved in. War is a pretty crappy thing to have to be sucked into. When I got back, I'd seen enough misery and cruelty that the only thing I wanted to pursue was beauty, and I found it in books. That's why I taught literature and didn't want to look back."

"Ever think about going back to teaching?"

"I'm content where I am right now. I don't miss the faculty meetings and deadlines for grades and kissing up to the higherups, and I have plenty of time for reading and thinking. I may even do a little writing myself. What about you? Do you have any ideas about a direction for yourself? You're a pretty bright guy. You could expand yourself. Is the doc giving you any ideas?"

"He's kind of pointed me a little in the direction of doing some kind of investigative work, but I would need to find some connection to someone who would trust me enough to do that kind of work for them. In the meantime, I thought I might try to connect with some of these student protest organizations just to find out what I can about them and how they work. It would be good practice and it would be interesting."

"Be careful, my friend, you don't want to get caught up in something that is going to land you in trouble. Some of these characters are pretty radical."

Meanwhile across town:

Fred had not moved in with Wanda and Maria, but he spent a lot of his time there. They had finished dinner and Wanda was preparing Maria to get ready for bed. She thought the time was right to tell her that her biological father was having a good success with the treatment for his leukemia and was almost ready to go back to his job. She told Maria that Fred had been helpful in finding someone who was a good match for the marrow donation.

Maria beamed at Fred and said, "Thank you, Fred. You are a good doctor."

Wanda said, "When you say your prayers tonight, say one for your dad, and don't forget to include Fred."

Maria smiled at Fred and gave him a big hug.

After Maria was in bed, Fred asked Wanda about the line of work Maria's father had been doing before he got ill.

"He was an investigative journalist for the paper. I guess he was digging into some of the financial interests of politicians and other rather shady people when he got ill. The leukemia apparently came on rather suddenly when his blood count suddenly dropped. They thought it was aplastic anemia at first, but then found some odd cell types in his blood and decided it was an unusual form of leukemia. His white count, platelets, and red cells all dropped rapidly, and the doctors feared that he would pick up a serious infection or have a serious bleed. They were glad that they found a donor when they did."

Fred smiled and said, "At some point, he might be interested in meeting his donor. If that happens, I could probably track Clarence down. I've run into him several times since he left the hospital, and I would probably be able to find him. It might be an interesting encounter, and it would probably be good for Maria's father to know of Clarence as a resource, in the event that he might need another marrow transplant in the future."

Wanda nodded and said, "That's a good thought, Fred. I can mention it to Jack and his wife and find out if he is open to the idea. Maybe you could bring it up to Clarence when you get the chance, and we'll see where it goes."

Fred had just seen Clarence in the office about a week before and wasn't scheduled to see him again for a couple of weeks. At their last appointment, Clarence had spoken to Fred about some of his experiences hanging out with some of the graduate students he had met at a bar and befriended. They took him for a student as well and invited him to join them at one of their SDS meetings, leaving Clarence with a feeling as though he were going to be acting like an undercover agent. Fred had warned him not to get too entangled in things that might get him in trouble. Though the hospital was not asking the police to pursue him, he had eloped and was an "escapee", and if he got in trouble, he might end up back on 2E. Fred was convinced that would not be in the best interests of Clarence, since he had expanded his world view and deflated his fears enough to not need hospitalization. He had made considerable personal growth in his contacts with Wilfred and others and was moving in the right direction using outpatient therapy. So far, he was making reasonably good choices, and his paranoia had subsided considerably. However, Fred reminded himself that Clarence had looked reasonably calm in the past and turned a field trip into quite a topsy-turvy event when his paranoia flared. Fred was glad that Clarence would be checking in with him on a somewhat regular basis.

Chapter 31:
UNDERCOVER EXPERIMENT

Clarence finished with his job at the library and knew that Wilfred was working on a special project that would keep him late into the evening. He decided to stop by a local pub to grab a bite to eat and a beer. The library job was beginning to bore him. It was not very stimulating, and Dr. Q. had put a bug in his ear about finding a career that would be interesting and might merge well with some of his skills. That kind of job might actually be enjoyable much of the time.

Walking into the pub, Clarence spotted a couple of graduate students he had met a week or so before over beers. They waved at him and invited him to join them.

"Hey Karl, haven't seen you in a week or so. Working hard on that poetry project?"

Clarence was still careful to use his alias. He had led them to believe that he was a graduate student in literature. They were both studying political science and history. Clarence thought literature was safe, since, if he needed to look more knowledgeable, he always had Wilfred to fall back on.

"Yeah, I had a paper to write and had to do quite a bit of research on it. Took a lot of time. Glad to be finished with it. What have you guys been up to, anything exciting? Anything new on the Cal State Fullerton situation?"

"We were just talking about that. In fact, we were just on our way to a meeting at a friend's apartment not too far from here to talk about it. Care to join us?"

"Sure, if that's Okay with whoever else would be there. Do you think there would be something cold to drink there? I was dying for a beer when I came in."

"Oh, I'm sure there will be plenty of refreshments there. Chauncey, the guy who is having the get-together usually has some appetizers, and there is usually a community pot bowl if you are interested. He makes some very good mushroom bruschetta sometimes. There will be a lot of people there who want to talk about the war. Come on along."

They left the bar and ambled down the street to what looked like an old fraternity house that had lost favor with the university. It had been converted into room rentals with a couple of large common rooms. They walked in to find a group of about twelve people in one large common room, some smoking pot, some drinking beer, and all talking about the war and how President Nixon was handling it. Clarence was introduced to Chauncey, who barely gave him a second glance, then continued his conversation with a couple of other grad students. It was easy for Clarence to meander around as though he were paying attention to various small groups of conversation and then moving on. He helped himself to a beer and congratulated himself on how he was able to eavesdrop without offering a lot of his own opinion. He saw a platter of crackers with a mushroom topping on the table and decided to try some. This must have been the mushroom bruschetta that his friends had mentioned. It was quite tasty, so he had a couple more, but stopped there. He did not want to look like he was just there to eat and drink, so he continued to wander from conversation to conversation.

Over the next half hour, Clarence had a growing sense of calm and peacefulness. He felt like he was floating along in the group, almost as though he were not walking but drifting like a log in the surf. He found it difficult to focus on the conversations as though what was being talked about was not, in fact, what was happening. Sounds began to take on color. Higher pitch voices were yellow; deep voices were blue or green; female voices were pink. Clarence saw a large dog at the entrance to the room. The pit bull seemed to be focused on him and bared its teeth. He looked away from it and saw it again in the fireplace, still staring at him. He became uneasy and asked a woman whose dog that was. She looked at him and said, "What dog?" Clarence was beginning to get frightened. He felt dizzy and nauseated. He decided to get the hell out of there, slipped out the front door and began to walk back to Wilfred's place. On the way back, he had the strong feeling that someone or several people were following him. He began to wonder if the mafia had picked up his trail and was ready to kill him. He had not worried about that threat for some time, but the fear was back. He took a round-about route to get home so that if they were following him, he might more easily spot them.

When he got to the apartment building, he sneaked around to the back door and let himself in. He kept the lights off so that no one would suspect there was anyone home. Clarence sat in the dark for what seemed like many hours. There was a little glow in the room from the streetlight outside, but vivid colors continued to appear with any little street noise such as cars going by or feral cats screeching. Clarence wondered if he was going crazy. While he sat as quietly as he could, he watched as two very large snakes slithered about the room until they found each other and began to twine around each other. One was quite red and the other a deep blue. They both looked at him. The red snake spoke to him in a female voice.

"Why do you fear us? We are you. We are your ancestors in you, but your ancestors are not you. We are you."

Pictures floated through his mind. He saw visions of children on skis in the mountains, of people in strange uniforms with weapons, of people running and falling. The visions went rapidly by but seemed at the same time to take forever. After a while Clarence began to get used to this kaleidoscope of images and the virtual cacophony of color. He became less fearful and more inquisitive. He seemed to be able to control the images by recalling photos that he had seen of Norway. Pleasant scenes took hold. He recalled as a child, his father coming to his room after he had a bad dream. In his memory, his father had kicked the monsters out of his closet and from under the bed and out the door of his room. Clarence laughed out loud at this memory.

The red snake spoke again. "You see, you need not fear. You can take control. Your ancestors are in you but do not control you."

It seemed like forever until Wilfred came home, but as Clarence found out eventually, it was only about two hours since Clarence had left work, gone to the bar, gone to the meeting, and had come home. When Wilfred entered and turned on the lights, he looked at Clarence and said, "What the hell are you doing sitting here all alone in the dark?"

"I was having an awful time. I was scared. I felt like the mafia was after me again. I'm having weird sensations and all kinds of strange things are happening."

"What the hell have you been eating? Did you get into some of that weird stuff that I warned you about?"

"I just went to a gathering of graduate students talking about the war and had a beer."

"Is that all? Did they give you anything else?"

"They had some crackers with some tasty mushroom sauce on top. I only had a few."

"They were probably magic mushrooms, the psychedelic kind. How many did you eat?"

"I just had a few."

"Looks like a few too many. It will probably take a while to wear off. Are you still having visions? That usually happens with that stuff. Lots of shamans among indigenous populations use similar plants or fungi to induce changes in perception to enhance religious or psychic experiences. Looks like the hippies have taken to it for different reasons, or maybe for some of the same reasons, given the war and the political scene. Let's turn the lights up and I'll make a pot of coffee. Maybe that will help settle things down for you."

Clarence was glad that the professor was there to help him through this experience. Time felt like it took forever to pass, and pieces of his life seemed to repeat themselves over and over, almost in slow motion. It was good to know that he was in the company of a safe person who was also a friend. For some reason the coffee, instead of making him more alert, seemed to calm him and make him drowsy, and he drifted off to sleep. He awoke in the morning to Wilfred making another pot of coffee.

"Good morning. Did you sleep it off? How do you feel? Ready for some coffee?"

As Clarence turned toward Wilfred's voice, it seemed as though it took a second for the room to catch up with his head turning, almost like those big loops that you dip into soapy water and wave to make a trailing bubble. It was like his senses had to catch up with his movement. This told him that he had not totally slept it off yet. It was good that today was Saturday, and he did not have to go in to work. It would take a while for him to make sense of his experiences of the night before and get his bearings again.

"Did I do anything strange after you got home last night?"

"No, after having a cup of coffee, you muttered something about dogs and snakes and lots of colorful noises, whatever that meant, but then you were dead to the world. Sounded like a weird experience."

Clarence went on to tell him about his experience the night before, the noises with color, the strange animals, and his sense of paranoia.

Wilfred listened patiently and said, "Those mushrooms, and whatever else they may have put in that stuff you ate, were probably the ones I warned you about -- 'magic mushrooms' that contain psilocybin, which is an hallucinogen commonly used by shamans in indigenous cultures for ceremonial or religious purposes. They tend to distort our perceptions and cause us to misinterpret our senses. This stuff can sometimes trigger emotions that are frightening or help us recall painful experiences, sometimes even things we have forgotten or pushed back deeply in our memories. The shamans would use these experiences to lead their followers into various beliefs or thought patterns or even a new tribal ethos. Lord knows what the hippies see in this stuff. Some of them go a bit crazy taking these things."

"How do you know all about this kind of stuff?"

"I have more time to read, and I have excellent access to books. I like reading about this kind of stuff. I've read enough poetry for a lifetime. I'm following Dr. Quimby's lead to explore other aspects of my life."

"These visions I saw last night were both frightening and piqued my curiosity. The snakes that I saw scared the shit out of me, but they seemed to be part of me somehow. They spoke to me like they knew me and knew my ancestors, and maybe were part of me and part of my ancestors at the same time. They seemed to want to keep us separate, but also connected. They wanted me to understand that my life was embraced by my family, but it is separate and belongs to me to live and shape. It was weird but electrifying in a way. It really jangled some nerves in me. They're still a bit jangled, but I don't think I want to let go of that underlying feeling of being connected but also separate and my own self."

"I would say that you should let the yeast cause the bread to rise for a while before you put it in the oven to bake. Know what I mean?"

"You mean think about it awhile before I use any more of those mushrooms or whatever else, right?"

"Right! It's got you thinking, now let the thoughts grow."

Chapter 32: COGITATION

Mushrooms don't take long to grow. All it takes is the right temperature and humidity and a forest floor with enough dead leaves and vegetation, and the spores will take root and pop up. Where there was nothing yesterday, today there may be scores of the little critters showing their caps. It just takes the right trigger to get the process going. So it was for Clarence. Whatever was in those party mushrooms seemed to be a catalyst for Clarence that allowed his emotional forest floor to be prepared to accept and cultivate what was coming his way. His readiness seemed to be tied to his upbringing and his family's history and culture, but his learning to face his fears enabled him to trust enough to form friendships. Suddenly, the timing was right, and he seemed ready to cultivate his experiences. Some would say it was luck, but to be able to take advantage of luck, one must be prepared to accept it and build on it. He was ready.

Clarence knew only a little of his family background. His parents didn't talk much about their time in Norway during the war before they migrated to the U.S. He didn't know his grandparents well. He was quite young when his parents came to the States. He knew a little about the war, but conversation about it generally was diverted when it came up in family conversation. Of course, he was aware that during World War II, the Germans had occupied Norway, but talking about that seemed to cause unease.

Clarence called his parents in hopes of having a real conversation. He first reached his mother. He reassured her that he was safe and had somewhere to live and had enough to eat. He told her that he had a job and a friend that he lived with. He checked to see if there had been any more inquiries about him, and there were not. He told her that he was comfortable and happy and generally reassured her. Then he asked to speak with Dad.

The conversation with his father was similar at first, reassuring him that he was OK and surviving well. After several rounds of reassurance, he said, "Dad, some things have come up for me that have made it important for me to know more about what things were like for you and Mom during the war and the Nazi occupation. I have these vague memories of photos, and I don't recall you or Mom ever talking much about your early years in Norway. What was Grampa's job during the war? How did you experience that time in your life?"

There was a long pause before his father answered. "Those were very tough years. We don't like to go back over those times and don't like to talk about it, but if it is important to you and your health, I'll try to answer any questions you might have about that time."

"What was it like? Was food rationed? Were people hurt or killed? You were probably young, but what did Grampa and Grandma do during that time?

"Food was hard to come by. The Germans confiscated a lot of things and sent them back home. We tried to raise basic things like potatoes and cabbage in our own gardens and tried to raise chickens and pigs when we could. There was a Resistance, but there were informants, too. As a result, numerous Resistance members were caught and shot. Your grandfather was part of the government, but when Quisling was appointed to lead the Norwegian puppet government, your grandfather was forced to continue his work there, and that angered many of our friends and neighbors. Most of our countrymen never discovered that he was secretly a part of the Resistance. He had to keep his role secret to be effective, and by the end of the war, most of the people whom he had been spying with, were dead.

After the war when the occupation ended, our family was shunned by most people, and my father had a very hard time earning enough for our family to get by. I was eighteen years old by that time. I met your mother, whose family did not want her to have anything to do with me. We fell in love. You know how it is when someone tells you not to have anything to do with someone you love. We managed to escape Norway by going to Sweden and then to England, and finally got to the U.S., where we eventually became citizens.

I continued to write to my parents after leaving, but I got word in 1948 that they had both died in an accident. The details of the accident were never clear, and I haven't been able to find out more. Because of the distortion of my father's reputation, we wanted to keep a low profile over the years, and we never really talked much about this with anyone, even our friends."

"So, Grampa was really a patriot! He was in the Resistance. He wasn't really working for Quisling."

"Yes, but most of his cohorts were killed by the Germans, so it never came out after the war about how much he had served to destabilize the occupiers by spying for the Resistance, using his government position."

Clarence had never really had a heart to heart with his father in all these years. This conversation was a totally new experience for him, and it saddened him to hear how his parents missed the last years with their own parents in order to be able to have a life for themselves. He thanked his father for speaking with him about the family and reassured him that he would be visiting soon, since he was now more settled in a new life for himself.

After hanging up the phone, Clarence thought back about his "mushroom trip". He could see that pieces of it began to make some sense, especially the part about the snakes talking to him. "Why do you fear us? We are you. We are your ancestors in you, but your ancestors are not you. We are you. You see, you need not fear. You can take control. Your ancestors are in you but do not control you."

The images were there, but he was no longer afraid. It was like putting a puzzle together. It would take some time.

Chapter 33:
THE DONOR CONNECTION

It was toward the end of March when Fred Quimby came to the library looking for Clarence. He asked Wilfred whether Clarence was still working there or living with him. He wanted to tell Clarence that the man to whom he had donated his marrow had made a complete recovery and wanted to meet his donor. Wilfred was happy to see Fred, and after they spent some time catching up, he quickly arranged for Clarence to connect with Fred.

It had been a few weeks since Clarence had been to the clinic to see him, and he had missed their last session. Clarence was surprised that Fred seemed to have tracked him down.

"Sorry, Dr. Q., I must have spaced out about our last session."

"Clarence, I'm not here about that. Remember the man who received your marrow donation? He seems to be doing quite well and is on the mend. He works as an investigative reporter for the newspaper and would like to meet with you and to thank you."

Clarence was intrigued that the marrow recipient was in that line of work. His curiosity aroused; he was eager for Fred to arrange the meeting happen.

"I would like to do that Dr. Q. You can either contact me here at the library, or at our next visit. I'm sorry I missed our last one, but I will call and set up another. By the way, I called my parents recently and had a nice conversation with them and found out some interesting family history that has got me thinking about things. We can talk about that at my next visit as well."

"I am glad to hear that, and I am glad that you are interested in meeting the man who got your marrow. I'll follow up with that and arrange a time for a meeting with him. Meanwhile, I hope the secretaries can fit you in for a session soon. But for now, I had better let you get back to work, and likewise for me."

Fred ambled off out the door.

Clarence was intrigued with the possibilities.

Chapter 34: ER DUTY

It was Saturday night, and Fred had pulled on-call duty at the emergency room. All the residents at the University Hospital pulled a stint there in rotation, under the supervision of a staff psychiatrist. Residents were the first in the line of action in the triage system. If someone came into the ER in need of psychiatric care, the resident was called first to determine the extent of the problem and whether medication or hospitalization would be needed. If so, the resident would then call the staff physician, discuss the issues, and be given the Okay to proceed with what needed to be done. Basically, the resident did the grunt work.

Saturday night in the University Hospital ER was often busy. Students were out and about taking advantage of the weekend, and overdoses on a variety of substances were not uncommon. Early in the evening, Fred was called to see a man who claimed to be a teenager but looked older, perhaps in his late 20's. He was being aggressive and was subdued on a gurney with his hands and feet held down with straps. He was screaming, spitting, and fighting the restraints. Fred recognized him as soon as he entered the room. It was Jack, the teenage alter of the patient at the state hospital whom he had treated for the dissociative disorder. Jack had come out of his imposed slumber.

"Jack, remember me? I am Dr. Quimby. We met at the other hospital. I am here to help you. How did you end up here?"

"Screw you, Quimby! The last time I talked to you, I fell asleep for a couple of months. When I woke up, I was still stuck in the hospital, but I fixed that. I just waited for the right time and slipped out."

"But how did you end up here? Did you lose track of time? Did you just wake up here?"

"No, I woke up in a convenience store trying to get something to eat, and when someone tried to get rough with me, I took out my knife and told him to back off. He called the cops. That's how I got here."

"Are you still hungry? I could probably get you something to eat, but you would have to settle down a lot before they would let me do that."

"Can I have a burger and fries?"

"I'll see what I can do about that. Can you settle down? Meanwhile while we're getting food, do you want something to drink, like milk or juice?"

"Juice would be really good, Doc."

"Have you had any contact with any of the others? Peter or Randolph, or Jonathon? The last time I spoke with any of them, they were trying to set up some lines of communication so everyone would know what was going on with the others. That way they could keep things straight and generally stay out of trouble."

"Well, sometimes that worked and sometimes it didn't. I hung on for a while, but I finally found a way to get out of the hospital. Then somewhere along the line, I lost track of things and ended up here in this hospital."

"Well, I think that was the whole idea: working together and keeping track of what was going on with all of you, so some of you didn't do things on your own, making it tough on everyone in the group, including yourself."

An attendant entered the room with a glass.

"Oh, here is your juice, but I am told the grill is closed and can't make hamburgers or fries, so they are sending a chicken salad sandwich over here in just a few minutes with some grapes on the side. Maybe once you have eaten, you can rest while I speak with Randolph."

When the sandwich came, an orderly loosened one arm to allow Jack to eat. He calmed down once his hunger was satisfied.

"You really look tired from all that excitement, Jack. Why don't you relax and let Randolph come to talk with me?"

He leaned back on the gurney and closed his eyes. A few seconds later, they opened again, and a calm voice said,

"Well, hello, Dr. Quimby. It's been a while. It looks like we have been on a safari from the other hospital for some time chasing wild beasts. I hope we have not been caught poaching or worse."

"Randolph, I am afraid Jack has managed to stir up a fuss, so you may end up on a police hold here in this hospital, or you may end up being transferred back to the other one. I hope the doctor in whose care I left you has worked out reasonably well for you. If they don't send you back there, you may end up stuck with me again in this place for a while."

"We were slowly making some headway with Dr. Mumbley. At least that's what I call him. He doesn't enunciate well, but he pretty much follows the guidelines you left for him. I wouldn't mind staying here and catching up with you if things work out that way."

"So, catch me up a little. I had met Jack and you and Peter as well as Jonathon. How many other characters pop out of hiding when they are needed? Or when they just sort of automatically take over? I know there are probably a few more."

"Well, Doc, Jonathon still doesn't know about all the others. Peter is like the little puppy who rolls over and whimpers, and people tend to leave him alone or try to take care of him. Jack is the angry teenager who has never really grown up. He thinks he is fending off danger, but he tends to cause most of the problems. Me, I am just the one who kind of hooks things together. There are a couple more that don't show up often. One is Annie, who is the sensitive one. She will show up sometimes when there is a lot of emotion welling up. She does a lot of crying and tends to clam up. Then there is Donald, who tries to keep all emotion bottled up and tries not to show any feelings."

"It sounds like Jack is the thorn in the side of all of you. How old was Jonathon when Jack showed up?"

"Well, he showed up about five years ago when Jonathon was in his twenties. He was acting like a 15 or 16-year-old when he arrived, and he hasn't changed much as far as maturity goes. He is still the same explosive teenage know-it-all."

"Maybe we could use the same method to help him grow up that we used to put him to sleep for extended periods of time. We can't just keep putting him to sleep. You are all part of the puzzles You all need to recognize that you are all pieces of the same person, but just taking turns trying to work different strategies to protect yourselves. Once that happens, we may be able to get you an unentangled life. Let's bring Jack back out so I can work with him."

Randolph put his head on his chest, closed his eyes, and seemed to sleep.

When his eyes opened, they quickly scanned the room.

Fred spoke first.

"Hi, Jack. Did you have a nice rest? Feeling better? You have been asleep a long time. You have had two birthdays since you dozed off. You are a veritable Rip Van Winkle.

"A who?"

"A Rip Van Winkle. He was a character in a story who went to sleep and woke up twenty years later. So, do you feel any older? You look like you have filled out well. You have matured quite a bit. Now that you are older, you will have much better control of your temper, and that should be a big help to keep you out of trouble. You will be able to think things through and find smarter ways to deal with things around you. But you still look tired, and I bet you could rest a bit more. In fact, it looks like you can barely keep your eyes open, and that's Okay, because you need the sleep. While you're sleeping, I'll be talking to Randolph for a bit. So, go ahead and get some well-needed sleep. I will see you again, but it may be a while --- maybe after another birthday."

Jack closed his eyes and put his chin on his chest. After a moment, the eyes opened again.

"Hello again Randolph. We will have to see if maturity comes with age. I have been told that you have been gone long enough from the State Hospital that you will be staying here at University Hospital for a while on a hold placed by the police. I have some calls to make and paperwork to do, but I will likely see you tomorrow. Let's see if we can keep Jack's siesta going through the night, and when I see him again, he will perhaps have aged another one or two years."

The patient was admitted to the psychiatric unit at University Hospital and Fred wrote the admission orders, which included a sedative, in case any of the alters got out of control. Fred would call the resident at the State Hospital on 2E to inform him of what had transpired here at the University Hospital.

Chapter 35: A BUSY WEEK

Once the weekend on call was over, it was back to the ward for Fred. He had to deal with the patient he referred to privately as "Terry and the Pirates", aka, Jonathon Maxwell. He planned to see Clarence in the outpatient clinic on Wednesday, so he was in the process of arranging a get-together with Clarence and Maria's father, Ronald Torkensen. All this was in addition to his regular patients and ward duties.

He started out Monday morning with Jonathon. He found Randolph still in charge.

"Well, how did the rest of the weekend go, Randolph?"

"Everybody has been quiet. They seem to know that we are safe here. Jack is still sound asleep."

"I think it is time for me to speak with Jack again. I need to reassure him that he is growing up. Will you please gently awaken him?"

Randolph put his chin on his chest and closed his eyes.

When he opened them again, they scanned the room again.

"Good morning, Jack. Did you sleep well?

"I slept like a log, Doc. How about you?"

'I slept and awakened many times since we last spoke, Jack. You were up to your Rip Van Winkle tricks again. You have had two more birthdays. You are now twenty years old; a grown man, mature and smart. I think you are ready to help solve the puzzle."

"What puzzle are you talking about, Doc?"

"Well, you know how it is sometimes when you are sleeping, it feels like you are dreaming about other people who are in charge of you? Well, these other people are all part of you. They have different ways of approaching problems that come up. Those ways are different than how you would tackle those problems. It's like you are all puzzle pieces. We have to put those pieces together so you can all see the whole picture and can work together in the same body and mind to get things done without getting into trouble. The best way I know to do that is for you to be especially aware when someone else is in charge. Watch them, understand why they are doing what they are doing, and when you don't understand it, ask one of the others or the doctor who is working with you. It will take some time, but you are a grown man, and you will be able to do it."

"That's a lot to soak in, Doc."

"It will take time and practice, but you are now mature enough to do it. Now, I want to let you get back into a sleep mode so you can observe and practice. So, let me speak with Randolph again please."

Jack put his chin on his chest, closed his eyes and slept. When his eyes opened again, Fred could tell it was Randolph.

"Hello again, Randolph. We'll just have to see how this goes for a while. I'll be checking on you at least daily while you are in this hospital. Any questions before I make my rounds on the unit?"

"We will see how it sinks in, Doc. Hope it works."

Fred went about his rounds. Over the next couple of days, he worked with Jonathon Maxwell's gang of pirates. Then the call came to send them back to the State Hospital. Fred called the 2E resident and filled him in about his approach. It sounded good on paper, but it would take a lot of time and work. The resident seemed eager to get at it.

Wednesday afternoon was outpatient day for Fred, and he was pleased to see that Clarence was again on his schedule. Clarence was eager to get at it. He started out talking about his contacts with the university students and their anti-war culture, but he quickly got into his experience with the hallucinogens. The colors, the mixing of senses, sounds having color, the dog, and the snakes talking to him seemed to have opened a Pandora's box of emotions and excitement. He especially wanted to know what Quimby thought of the snakes and their words.

"Clarence, snakes have a prominent place in ancient and in indigenous cultures. They are mysterious with a magical context and have a symbolism of healing, because they shed their skins. They have a place in medicine in many ancient stories. The caduceus is a medical symbol that came about when the Greek god Hermes broke up a fight between two snakes by throwing his winged staff at them. They wound themselves around it, forming the caduceus. Interestingly many shamanistic cultures that use hallucinogens also focus on snakes, often visualizes as intertwining together, like the double helix of DNA. In your case, it looks like the snakes you saw, though frightening at first, seemed to be reassuring you that no matter where you came from, or what experiences you have emerged from, you have the opportunity to become yourself."

"I did have some contact with my parents by phone, and I found out a lot about my family history."

Clarence filled Fred in about the conversation he had with his father about the war, his grandfather's role in the resistance, and his parents' reticence to talk about it much as he grew up.

"It looks like your parents' reluctance to engage people sort of rubbed off on you. Now that you know more about them and their circumstances, it can free you up to be who you want to be. It seems to have given you a new infusion of energy. Speaking of energy, the man to whom you donated your marrow has gained a lot of energy and wants to meet you to thank you. I have arranged for that to happen. All we have to do is to come up with a time and place. Let's work that out."

They put their heads together and Fred said he would make it happen. They spent the rest of the hour going over more of the insights that Clarence had sorted out on his own. Fred had seen Clarence animated before, but his energy and excitement was at a different level today. Fred wondered how much longer Clarence would need to be coming back to see him. He guessed it would be a few more times before the need dropped off.

Chapter 36:
TEMPUS FUGIT
July 1972

Fred Quimby had finished his psychiatry training in 1972. Because of the Viet Nam war and, as a newly minted psychiatrist, he had an obligation to enter the military. Several of his cohort were sent to Viet Nam or bases that served as catchment areas for survivors who were returning. Fred was sent to fight the Russians in the cold war. In other words, he was sent to a missile base in the western U.S. There he spent his time dealing with G.I.'s, both drafted and enlisted men, many of whom were not thrilled to be in military service. By this time, Fred and Wanda had been married about two years and Marie was almost nine years old. Fortunately, since they were stateside, Fred could bring his family with him.

Fred arrived by car at his base in Montana as ordered, without having gone through basic training. Apparently, there was an immediate need for a psychiatrist at this base, so he arrived in civilian clothes. He had driven alone to get there because he had yet to obtain housing. Wanda and Marie planned to fly out to join him once he was assigned living quarters.

At the base gate, he was stopped by security police until he explained his purpose for being there and why he was not in uniform. He presented his orders, and then was directed to the base hospital. It was a small hospital as hospitals go. Fred found his way to the emergency room and spoke to an airman who was on duty. The airman spoke to his superior, who in turn called the colonel. The colonel arrived, looked him up and down and said, "Where is your uniform?"

"I'm sorry, sir, I don't have one."

"Didn't you get one at basic training?"

"I haven't been to basic training, sir."

"What do you mean? Everyone here goes to basic training."

"My orders told me to go directly to my assigned base and not to go to basic training. I got the impression that I was badly needed here." Fred handed him the orders he was sent.

The colonel looked at the orders and frowned. He looked at a young lieutenant standing nearby. "Lieutenant Jones, take this man to the BX and get him into a uniform. Then bring him back to my office so I can acquaint him with what goes on here in the hospital and what his duties will be."

So off they went to the Base Exchange. Lieutenant Robert Jones helped him to obtain a summer uniform and suggested the rest of the uniform could come later. Then he brought Fred to his own off base home to meet his wife, Helen. Jones asked Helen if she could hem the pants of Fred's uniform for him on her sewing machine. Fred and Helen exchanged niceties and she went straight to her Singer. When she had finished sewing, she said to Fred, "When your family gets to the base, I would be more than happy to show your wife around town and fill her in a little about military life."

Fred thanked her. "She will be more than happy to have someone here who can help her with that. Thanks, she'll be in touch. Meanwhile, may I use your bathroom to change into my new uniform that you so kindly tailored for me?"

She smiled and pointed to the bathroom. The uniform fit nicely. Fred came out and smiled at her and said, "Thank you very much for the extra trouble."

She smiled back and said, "No trouble at all, Dr. Quimby."

He said, "Just call me Fred."

Then Jones brought him back to the base to meet with the colonel again.

"Here he is sir. All set to go. We just started with his summer uniform for now."

"Good job, lieutenant. At least it's a beginning. Let's show him his office and the rest of the hospital."

They walked to the psychiatrist's office, which was a room off a hallway, beyond which were the offices of ob-gyn and pediatrics. The psychiatry office consisted of two rooms, one for his corpsman, who would answer the phones and keep his schedule, and one for him to see patients. Fred's space had a desk, a couple of chairs, a small closet, a file cabinet, and a phone. There were chairs in the hallway for his patients to wait.

The colonel said, "We see both active-duty personnel and their dependents here. Your corpsman will make appointments for you, so you can work that out with him. I will leave it up to Lieutenant Jones to show you around the rest of the hospital, the mess hall, surgery suites, and so on. You have already been to the ER. Like all the doctors here, you will take your turn on call in the ER as medical officer of the day. I am sure your helper, Airman Pride here, will be able to acquaint you with some of the routines in your section. If you have further questions, you can check with me later."

Fred said, "I do have one question, colonel – where do I sleep tonight, and when will I have quarters for me and my family when they arrive? I can't send for them until we have a place to live."

"Oh, you will stay in the officers' quarters, but we should be able to assign you a house within a couple of days, and then you can have your belongings shipped here. You should be able to have your family settled in here in a week or so. Lieutenant Jones can direct you to the officers' quarters."

With that brief introduction, the colonel walked away. Fred watched him leave and then turned to meet Airman Pride, his new assistant. Fred reached out to shake his hand and introduced himself. They spoke briefly about what his hours would be; then he turned to Lieutenant Jones and said, "I don't want to keep you from your job. Perhaps you can show me where I will be staying for the time being. Then I will come back later and go over the job here with Airman Pride."

Lieutenant Jones looked at him and said, "You are my job right now, sir. When I am done with you, I'll have to go back and hang around the colonel to see what he wants me to do next. Let me show you around the base. There is really not much for you to do in your office today except to acquaint yourself with the job, and you have all day tomorrow learn the ropes. After I show you around, we can stop by the Officers Club. You will need to get to know that place."

They did a quick tour of the rest of the hospital followed by a ride around the base to see the airfield, the housing units, and the NCO club. They stopped at the administration building. There they got him officially signed into the base, got his pay set up, and arranged for his security clearance. They finally got to the Officers' club and ordered beer. They spent a leisurely hour over brews and talking about the military. Then Lieutenant Jones, who was by now Bob, felt it would be a good idea to get Fred to his quarters and get him checked in. It was a single room with a single bed, a small dresser, a miniature closet, a small mirror and a sink. The common shower and bathroom was down the hall.

Fred's car was parked near the hospital, so he returned there with Bob and decided he had best get better acquainted with Airman Pride and get the lay of the land. He wanted to check to see what his schedule would be for the following day. After that he could return to his room with his other belongings that were stashed in the trunk of his car.

It was by now close to five in the afternoon when Fred returned to his office in the hospital. Airman Pride was still there.

"I am glad I caught you still here, Airman Pride. What is your first name if you don't mind?"

"It's William, sir, but I go by Bill."

"Is it OK with you if I call you Bill? You can call me Dr. Q. or Fred if it doesn't get you funny looks around here."

"Sounds good to me, Doc."

"You're working a little late. When is quitting time around here?"

"I'm on duty till midnight today, sir. My duties require me to be on the lookout for spies and saboteurs till then. Have you seen any spies or saboteurs, sir?"

"No, I can't say that I have."

"Well, see what a good job I am doing?"

Fred knew he would get along with Airman Pride just fine.

"Look Doc, you don't have to stick around. There is nothing on the schedule so far for tomorrow. I can fill you in on the details in the morning. I will be here at 0800, but you won't need to get here till about nine. That's probably about when the colonel will be nosing around to check on you. As far as meals, you can get breakfast at the mess hall if you get there before 8:30 and lunch is available between 11:30 and 1:00. You are probably best off getting dinner at the Officers' Club or at the little steakhouse that's just off base. I presume Lieutenant Jones arranged for a place to sleep until you get your regular quarters."

Fred left the hospital and went to his car. After dropping his gear at his assigned room, he decided to check out the steak house. He drove out the gates and past the outdoor movie theater featuring 'Slaughterhouse Five' to arrive at the Buckaroo Steakhouse. He had the best ribeye steak he had ever eaten, paid the bill and drove back to the base to find a telephone, so he could call Wanda and Marie to tell them about his first day in the Air Force.

Chapter 37:
GETTING USED TO THINGS

Fred got acquainted with his office and his duties over the next few days. He hit it off well with airman Pride. His main tasks were to see airmen who were having difficulty adjusting to military service and adhering to rules and protocols. He also saw some dependents, namely wives who had to hold down the fort at home while their husbands were out to the missile sites scattered over hundreds of miles. There were also people who were retired from the service who needed to be followed by a physician. Since there were no VA hospitals in the area, they were allowed to come to the base hospital for care. Then there were those airmen who were sent to see the psychiatrist, because their commanders did not know what else to do with them.

Since Fred had not been to basic training, he had not received the various vaccines that all military personnel received upon their reporting for duty. He talked to the pharmacy technician about getting them. The tech, in turn, said he would check into it and make the necessary arrangements.

Several days went by, and not having heard anything more about the shots, he again spoke to the pharmacy tech.

"Have you made any arrangements about my shots?"

The tech answered him saying, "It's all taken care of, Doc."

"So, when do I come in to get them?"

"Like I said, Doc, it's all taken care of."

"But don't I need to come in and……"

"Doc, it's all taken care of."

Fred got the gist of things sometimes being taken care of differently in the military.

A few days later, Fred had his first turn at spending time in the ER as medical officer of the day. His duties included dealing with medical issues other than psychiatry. During the day, he was approached by the Ob-Gyn doctors who told him that they had a woman who might well go into labor. They would be busy with a complicated surgery, and if she did go into labor, he would need to scrub in and handle the delivery for them. Not having scrubbed in for a delivery in over three years, Fred gulped a bit but said he would be ready.

Sure enough, about three in the afternoon, he was called to the delivery room. He quickly got into scrubs and began scrubbing his hands for the delivery. He gloved up, but she was moving fast. He got ready just as the head was crowning and caught the little guy, handed him to the nurse, got the cord cut and waited to deliver the placenta. He looked at the mother, handed her the baby and said, "There ma'am, now you can tell everyone that the base psychiatrist delivered your baby."

She smiled and said, "Oh thank you, I will."

Fred was relieved that it went so quickly that he did not have to do an episiotomy.

That evening Fred was still on duty in the ER. A young lieutenant was brought in by a friend. He had a gunshot wound to the leg. The story was that he had been practicing quick draw with a .22 caliber revolver and inadvertently pulled the trigger before the gun was out of the holster and shot himself in the leg. Fred didn't question the details of the story. He made sure any bleeding was stopped and then got in touch with one of the surgeons to check out the wound and treat it.

Soon afterward, a call came in requesting a helicopter be sent to one of the missile sites about three hundred miles from the base to pick up a man who had fallen and hurt himself. Fred investigated and learned that a chopper could not be sent out that late at night, because there would not be enough light to be able to safely land at the remote site. Fred had to deal with the issue over the phone and to make sure the injured airman would be Okay until morning. All in all, when he went off duty the next morning, he hoped all his MOD times were not a hectic as this.

Fred was relieved to be assigned housing and arranged for a moving company to bring the family furniture and other belongings to the base. The van was to be arriving the next day, and Wanda and Marie could then fly out to join him as well. Anticipating their arrival helped with his loneliness. He had met a few of the docs, but some of them were finishing up their tours and getting ready to depart. New arrivals were expected, but their time was also taken up by orienting to a new life. After his on-call stint, he checked with Airman Pride at the office, but nothing was scheduled, so he left the hospital to get some sleep. He decided to check out his new housing on the way. Since he planned to call Wanda that evening, he thought it would be nice to tell her a little about it. It was not anything fancy, but it should work well. The house had two bedrooms and a bathroom upstairs and a living room, a dining area, and kitchen downstairs with a laundry area just off the garage. It would do just fine for them.

Chapter 38:
ARRIVAL OF THE INNOCENTS

A little over a week passed before Fred picked up Wanda and Marie at the local airport. Fred had driven them through town a bit before getting to the base, so they could get a general idea of the community. It was not a big town, but it had a mall, some restaurants, pleasant looking neighborhoods, a downtown area, a library, a local hospital, and schools. Then they went to the base where the airmen at the gate saluted Fred as they drove in. They took a quick loop around the base, and Fred pointed out what he could. They arrived at their living quarters. Fortunately, the furniture had been delivered a couple of days before, and Fred had been able to get the beds and furniture set up, and the dishes put away, so when they arrived, it had some resemblance of order. They would have to buy groceries, but tonight they would eat out.

They walked through the house, checking out what was where, then sat around their new living room and filled each other in about their adventures of the last two weeks. Wanda and Marie had stayed with friends and generally had a nice time while Fred was adjusting to being in military service.

Fred looked at them and said, "I missed you both a lot, but I have been very busy getting used to the new job and getting things ready for your arrival. We will still have stuff to unpack and get ready, and I will need to find out about school in the fall and how to get the two of you acquainted with people, but you are both probably hungry, so let's get to a restaurant and get a bite to eat."

Wanda said, "I am famished. How about you, Maria?"

"There is a great steakhouse right outside the base. What say we go there, and we can talk all we want while we eat?"

They dashed to the car and drove to the Buckaroo Steakhouse, where they spent the next couple of hours eating, laughing, and catching up.

When they got ready to go, Maria went over to the waitress and said, "Thank you. That was the most delicious hamburger I have ever tasted, and your suggestion about the rhubarb pie made my day." The waitress grinned.

When they got back to the house, they unpacked, rearranged some of the furniture, and more or less got settled. Maria found her books and made sure she stashed them in what would be her bedroom. By this time, she was bushed and was ready to go to bed. Fred and Wanda caught up some more, waited for Maria to go to sleep, then went to bed themselves and caught up some more.

The next morning, Fred walked to the hospital, which was not that far, and he left the car with Wanda so she could get some groceries Wanda wanted to check in with the local nursing association in the area to see if there was anything she needed to regarding licensure, in case she had an opportunity to work.

When Fred got to his office, he had a patient waiting. It was a military policeman who had been sent in by his CO for an evaluation of his fitness for duty. He was a man in his mid-twenties who said he had recently returned from Viet Nam.

He said, "Over in Nam, we were under fire, and no one was looking over our shoulder to see if our shoes were shined or whether our uniforms were on right. Here we are out in the middle of nowhere guarding missiles sites. If everything is calm and there is no excitement, we're doing a good job. If a rabbit or a deer sets off a sensor, all hell breaks loose, and we catch hell. If our uniforms aren't just right, we get written up. I lost my temper and said that to my sergeant. That's what got me in trouble. So, he sends me to the shrink to see if I am nuts."

Fred looked at him. "Are you nuts?"

"No, I'm not nuts, Doc. I'm just pissed. I'm bored stiff with this job. I have to be on site for a couple days at a time. I finally get to spend time with my wife and kid after a year in Nam, and now I'm gone most of the time and can't even see them at night until I get back to the base for a day, then it's back out to the boonies for another couple days."

"So how do you plan to deal with it?"

"I need to keep my cool and put in for a transfer to the motor pool or the flight line or something else."

"Do you think you can keep it cool?"

"Yeah, Doc, I can. I just had a bad day that day. I wasn't ever in trouble in the year I spent in Nam."

"Well, I will write a report that says that I find you sane and competent. It's up to you to do the rest. You do need to keep your temper in check. If they send you back to see me again, I probably won't be able to keep you out of hot water."

"OK, Doc, Thanks."

Fred excused him, and he left the office.

Fred checked with Airman Pride to find no one on the schedule for the next hour, so he went to the mess hall to get a cup of coffee and a snack. He saw a couple of other docs sitting at a table and wandered over. He had been introduced before, but it was an opportunity to get better acquainted. The other docs filled him in on some of the available distractions in town and on the base. There was a pool on base that families could use. There was a bus that took kids to school once it started up. The base also had a movie theater and a bowling alley for the long winters. The town had a library that military and families could use.

Sometimes some of the medical families would get together at different homes to let loose, but, best of all, some of the docs had a poker game every couple of weeks. With some of the docs finishing their tours and new ones coming on, there definitely would be room at the table for newcomers. Things were looking up already.

Chapter 39:
TEMPUS FUGIT AGAIN
September 1972

September arrived rather quickly. Marie made friends at the pool and started school in town, taking the base bus with her new-found friends. Wanda managed to connect with Helen Jones and with the wives of several of Fred's colleagues at the hospital. She was also able to get in contact with the licensing people and managed to get a part-time gig filling in at the local mental health clinic. New medical staff at the hospital were filtering in from basic training, and Fred had gotten to know them. They were from many different areas of the country and generally seemed to be a good bunch. Most of the new docs were "inductees" like himself.

As usual, Fred walked to the hospital from his house. He had gone home for lunch and was a little early returning to his office.

Airman Pride burst into the office and said, "Doc, quick, get to the ER. You're the only doc back from lunch, and they need you to take an ambulance out to the flight line immediately."

"Where is the MOD?"

"He's already out on the flight line with the other ambulance. Just get to the ER. They need a doc there right away."

Fred hurried and one of the corpsmen said, "Doc, just get in. Let's go." The ambulance took off for the flight line. When they arrived, they saw the other ambulance, a couple of corpsmen and a doctor. The medical personnel all had gas masks on, and several other people were lying around with small signs pinned to their chests. Another person, also unmasked, was walking around with a clipboard taking notes.

It was obviously a drill. Fred walked up to the other doctor, hoping to assess the situation. However, Fred saw the caduceus on his lapel but could not make out who it was. His gas mask was all clouded up, and Fred could not understand what he was saying through the mask. He obviously could not breathe well with the mask on and kept pulling the mask away from his face to take a few deep breaths. Fred, uncertain what to do next, began going around to check the signs on the chests of the victims. As the other ambulance began to load victims, Fred decided to start loading his own ambulance. Then the man with the clipboard lay down and put a sign on his chest that said, "heart attack". The corpsmen asked what to do with him, so Fred said, "Finish getting these other guys loaded up." When that was done and they asked Fred what to do about the clipboard guy, Fred said, "Throw him in there too."

They drove back to the base, and the corpsmen unloaded the victims of the drill. Fred then went to his office. A few minutes later the colonel came to his office.

"Dr. Quimby, you saved the day today."

"How so, Colonel?"

"When that inspector showed that he had a heart attack, and you put him on the ambulance last, we could take him off first when you got to the hospital. Because we got him off first, being the most urgent patient, we passed the inspection."

Realizing how fortuitous the circumstances had been, Fred smiled.

"Well, Colonel, when you send someone to do the job, you just have to send the right person."

"Well done, Doctor."

"Thanks, Colonel."

After he left, Fred breathed a sigh of relief. He was winging it all the way, out on that flight line.

Looking at his schedule for the afternoon, Fred saw one of his regulars would be coming in. It was Sergeant Bradley who had served for eighteen and a half years before being assigned to an ROTC unit in an east coast college. Apparently, there were a several cadets who were not keen on being in the military, but because it was a land grant college, at least a year of ROTC was required. Sergeant Bradley did not get along with several of these students, and there was enough friction that things managed to get physical. The result was that Sergeant Bradley was put on TDRL, which stood for Temporary Duty Retired List. Essentially, that meant that he was not on active duty and could not finish out his twenty years to retirement until he was able to return to active duty. Sergeant Bradley was essentially in limbo. Thus, he had to see a psychiatrist on a regular basis until he could be found fit to return to active duty or be discharged for medical reasons. Sergeant Bradley was from Montana, so he returned to live there and had been in to see Fred several times. He had a part-time gig at the local mall. The mall managers would arrange a "gunfight" periodically between two cowboys with six-shooters as a publicity stunt. One would call the other out and they would draw on each other shooting blanks. Sergeant Bradley was the one dressed in black who always got killed.

Sergeant Bradley was frustrated with being in limbo and would often go camping to get away. On one occasion, he was in his camper truck when a large group of "hippies" pulled up to the space next to his and started to play loud music. After a while, he asked them to keep the noise level down. They continued to cook dinner and turned the volume up a notch. Bradley went into his camper, got his .357 magnum, and, in his words, "shot a big hole right through their communal stew pot. They packed up and left. Things were quiet again."

A second incident also occurred while camping. He had made friends with another camper, when he heard on the radio that two men had escaped from prison. There was a description of the men and their vehicle. When another party arrived, he said to the man he had befriended, "I think those are the guys we heard about on the radio. You go get the sheriff and I will keep them here until you get back." He kept an eye on the two men, and at one point, when it looked as though they might get into their car and leave, he held them at gunpoint to wait for the sheriff. When they started to move toward their car, he shot at a branch over their heads that fell beside them. He yelled, "I said, don't move." When his friend came back with the sheriff, it turned out the two men were not the escapees. The pair quickly left the campsite.

Since Sgt. Bradley was on Fred's list again for the day, he thought about taking advantage of the situation. Patients had been uncomfortable with the waiting area. Fred began asking them what they thought of it. Most thought it was terrible. They would say things like, "I am waiting to see the psychiatrist for personal things and people are walking by to Ob-Gyn and Pediatrics. It should be more private."

Fred would mention that there was a suggestion box at the end of the hall, and maybe they could use it to bring up their concerns. After Sergeant Bradley's session, Fred mentioned the suggestion box.

"I'll do better than that. I'm going to go talk to the colonel!" And he stormed off to the colonel's office.

The following day, the head nurse came in to see Fred and closed the door behind her.

"Dr. Quimby, I was checking the suggestion box at the end of the hall. Do you know that out of twelve suggestions, eleven of them were about the waiting area for your office?"

"Really? Well, people have mentioned to me that it is uncomfortable sitting out there to wait for their appointments."

"Well, then, I think I will bring this up at our weekly meeting with the colonel."

The following day, a storage area was refitted to make space for a waiting room.

After Sgt. Bradley's trip to see the colonel, Fred was asked to write up a report regarding Sergeant Bradley's fitness for further duty, or if not, a recommendation for a release from TDRL. This, in turn, would allow a medical discharge from the service, with a pension. Fred recalled his father's favorite adage, "There's more than one way to skin a cat."

A few days later, Fred saw another medically retired sergeant who had been injured in an airplane accident while on duty. He was discharged from service because of his injuries and was given a pension based on his disability. He came in to see the base psychiatrist because he was depressed. He lived in Montana and had settled in town, but he could not work or he would lose his pension. Being unemployed, he sought every hobby he could to occupy himself. He purchased a rock polisher and tried to make different kinds of jewelry. He tried gardening. He tried canning different kinds of food. He tried weaving blankets. None of it lasted. He would become bored. He saw Fred and said,

"I'm a nervous wreck, Doc. I've tried every hobby I can think of and nothing lasts long. I'm starting to drink too much beer. I need something else."

Fred looked at him and said, "Do you like to fish? You've lived here a long time. You must know fishing and hunting places around here."

"Well, yeah, but my kid goes to school and my wife works, and I don't want to just go off by myself."

"OK, Sergeant Glide, your job is to take me to some good fishing spots, and when hunting season starts, we'll do that too."

Fred watched his eyes light up.

"All right, Doc. I'm going to start by taking you up to a place that was stocked with fish two years ago, but they just opened it to fishing this year. We're going to catch us some fish!"

About two weekends later, when Fred had time off, he arranged to rent a small tent trailer, brought poles and gear and headed with his patient and new-found guide, Frank Glide to northern Montana to a small pothole lake. They had planned to stay for a couple of days. They got set up and went down to bait up and catch some fish. Frank put a sinker at the end of his line, tied two dropper lines with bare hooks about a foot apart above the sinker, and opened a can of corn. He put a kernel of corn, a piece of worm and a miniature marshmallow on each hook. He cast the line out into the lake and sat back, and said, "Now we're fishing."

Fred looked at him and thought, "Good lord, we're going to be just sitting around for two days doing this?"

Fred half-heartedly started to set up his gear, but before he could get finished, Frank was chasing his pole as it was dragged down to the water's edge with a fish on.

They had filled up a large cooler with trout, between eleven and eighteen inches long, by the end of the day. There was no room to carry any more, so they slept in the tent, talked a lot about Frank's military experiences and family, and planned some future trips. They packed up the next day to go home. Frank took a few of the fish, but most in the cooler went to Fred. His house did not have a freezer, so Fred and

Wanda planned a fish fry for the staff at the hospital to come and eat barbecued trout.

Chapter 40:
TOUCHY BUSINESS
July 1973

Fred was aware that he had to follow the rules. One of his colleagues had pushed the limits in small but annoying ways. He was a flight surgeon with a three-year hitch compared to most of the other docs, who were in for two years. When he showed up to get his official photo taken, he was told that he would have to trim his mustache, that had grown below the corner of his mouth. He did so, but when he returned the following week to take the photo, his sideburns were too long, and he was told to trim them and come back. On the third trip, the picture showed that he had some food stuck to his teeth, so the picture had to be taken again. On the fourth try, he purposely combed his chest hair so that it came up over his collar. His next notification consisted of orders to go to Viet Nam.

Fred was also aware that the time when most young doctors finished their training was usually in early July. It was unlikely that they would easily find a replacement for him in a timely way if he were shipped off to another duty station. Unless he totally screwed up, he was reasonably safe in his present assignment. He felt a little emboldened by this thought, considering how they had originally rushed him to his duty station without basic training, because they had a scarcity in the psychiatrist pool.

Fred got back from lunch and was told that the Sergeant Major wanted to see him, so he sauntered down to his office. When he arrived, the Sergeant Major said, "Congratulations."

Fred said, "What did I do?"

"You have become a major."

"Well, I was just getting used to being a captain."

"Well, now you're up in rank to major."

"Okay, does that mean I get a raise?"

"Yes, I guess it does."

"How much?"

"I'm not sure."

"Can you look it up?"

The Sergeant Major looked in a large folder and said, "About $37 per month."

"That ought to be enough to buy the extra brass I'll need. Will I move from company grade housing to field grade housing?"

"Don't you like where you are living?"

"Well, yes, it's fine, but if I am going to be a major, I think I should be entitled to field grade housing."

"Yes, if you want field grade housing, I guess we can get you into some."

"Okay, is that it?"

"We just need you to sign something."

"What is it you want me to sign?"

"You just need to sign that you will continue to serve in the Air Force for two years from the point of your Majority."

"Whoa. I have just served for one year of a two-year hitch, and you want me to start over?"

"Well, those are the rules for promotion."

"I think I have a better idea. Why don't you just make me a lieutenant and let me out now?"

"Oh, come on, Doc, some guys would jump through all kinds of hoops to get this."

"Well, Sarge, Right now like I kind of like being a captain. I'm not ready to sign on for two more years as a major. Sorry."

Fred excused himself and walked out of the office. He went down to the medical supply office where another captain was in charge. He had come up through the ranks and had earned his rank the hard way. When Fred told John what had just transpired, he was aghast.

"Just tell them you'll take it if they will send you to Spain."

"If I did go to Spain or somewhere else overseas, I would have to put in three more years. No, thanks. I have one kid and Wanda is pregnant with another. I don't even know if they would let me bring them to wherever they might end up sending me. They sent you to Turkey, John. I have to consider my family."

John just shook his head. Fred could see that John would have loved to jump through those hoops to be able get another promotion.

Fred walked down the hall to his office.

The patient who was waiting to see him was a sergeant who had served for eighteen years. Fred had seen him a month previously for an urgent consultation requested by a fellow doc. Sergeant Gray had spent a tour in Viet Nam and was assigned to duty here at this base when he returned. He was proficient at his job, and the colonel who ran the base invited him to attend a meeting with a group of officers in charge of various key activities on the base. The colonel used the sergeant to demonstrate deficiencies in how these staff officers were running things, by asking him to contrast his experiences in such matters, essentially calling the officers on the carpet at the sergeant's expense. Obviously, this did not go over well with the officers involved, one of whom was in command of the administration building. The next thing Sergeant Gray knew, was that he received orders to go back to Viet Nam. Having just returned from a tour there, he began to go through channels to have the orders changed.

One thing led to another until he was admitted to the hospital prior to being sent off to Travis AFB the following morning for a thorough psychiatric assessment. The internist, who had admitted the sergeant to spend the night. He realized that something was fishy and called Fred and asked him to do an emergency evaluation that evening, so that Fred's opinion could go with the patient and his chart the following morning. Fred interviewed Sergeant Gray that evening in the hospital for two hours. He handwrote a report, which essentially said that it looked like the sergeant was being railroaded, that he was not mentally ill, that he was a capable military man, and that he should be returned to full duty. Fred made sure the report was placed into the sergeant's chart. The next morning, he and his chart were sent off to Travis.

About thirty days later, Sergeant Gray was back.

"I just wanted to thank you for helping me out before I was sent off to Travis, Doc. Your report was taken seriously. They kept me there to let things cool down up here before sending me back. When I got back, the colonel who put me in that meeting with those officers ended up getting a reprimand. He called me into his office to berate me, because he blamed me for his not getting promoted to general."

"What did you do?"

"I just did what I had to. I sat there until he was done ranting and then asked to be excused. I really want to thank you for going out of your way to come in and see me at night and putting in a good word for me. Thanks again, Doc."

Fred smiled, shook his hand, and said, "Good luck, Sarge. I hope this fiasco is all over now."

"I don't think they want to mess around with me anymore, not after the colonel got a reprimand. None of them want to take the chance that this might backfire on them any more than it already has."

With that, he saluted Fred and left the office.

Chapter 41:
WORKING THE SYSTEM

One day Fred had another sergeant's dependent wife come to see him. This woman was in her early forties, and her husband had been stationed at this base before being ordered to Viet Nam. Because of his assignment elsewhere, she could no longer live here on base, so with her four children, she moved to a small house just off base so that she could continue to use military services. Groceries were cheaper in the BX, and she could continue to use the medical services. She also thought her kids could take the school bus from the base to their school in town. The school bus access, however, was not allowed, because she lived "off base". Two of her children were in special education, and she was generally having a tough time. From her perspective, things were very bad, and she was at the point of seriously considering suicide. Fred saw her condition as a serious risk. He tried to work with her on an outpatient basis, but ultimately had to admit her to the hospital, where she could be monitored. She was able to get some relatives to come and care for the kids for a while, but after two weeks as an inpatient, Fred was getting some pressure to do something else.

Fred knew he had to get the husband back from Nam. An opportunity arose when he saw that the colonel was off base on business. Fred called the Red Cross. He told them that Sergeant Meyer had a wife who was seriously ill and needed to be sent back to the states to be with her.

A few days later, the colonel was back and was speaking to someone in the ER when he saw an ambulance getting ready to leave.

He asked the driver, "Where is that ambulance going?"

The driver said, "We're going to the city airport to pick up a GI. He apparently had a nosebleed from Salt Lake City to our airport, so they called us to pick him up."

"Where was he coming from?"

"They told us he was returning from Viet Nam."

"Who sent for him from Nam?"

"I think it was Dr. Quimby, sir."

The colonel turned to the lieutenant behind him and said, "Get Quimby to my office now."

When Fred got the word, he immediately went to the colonel's office.

"Good afternoon, sir." Fred could see that the colonel was fired up. He was taller than Fred, who noted the colonel's epaulet was sticking up from his collar.

"I understand that you sent for Sergeant Meyer from Viet Nam."

Fred said, "Excuse me, sir, your epaulet is out." He reached up to slip the material back under the colonel's collar. It gave him a moment to collect his thoughts, as the colonel blushed visibly at his own indiscretion. Fred remembered his encounter with Dr. Nolan a couple of years before. "Well, sir, the situation with his wife's suicidal intentions was serious. You were off base and unavailable, and I knew something had to be done, so I said to myself, what would colonel Polon do in a situation like this? And I knew that you would have said to call the Red Cross and get this guy home, so we could resolve this situation. So that is what I did."

The colonel pondered this reply for a moment, then said,

"Well, Dr. Quimby, I am happy to see that you thought it through and used good judgment in the situation. Let's see if we can't get this matter cleared up and get this lady back on her feet. I will see that there is a position on this base to put him to work while you work with his wife. Congratulations, Dr. Quimby. Well done."

"Thank you, sir. Will that be all for now?"

"Yes, Doctor, you are excused."

Fred nodded and left the room, breathing a sigh of relief as he walked toward his office. His time in the military kept had him on his toes, accommodating both the rules and regulations and the culture, but he had managed to keep his sense of self intact. He was grateful that he was able to have both Wanda and Maria here at his posting to keep him balanced. Both had made friends here. Maria was enjoying school and living in another part of the country, seeing it as an adventure. Wanda had found part-time work that kept her stimulated, and she had made some good friends among some of the other doctors' wives. Fred had also made some good friends among the docs and some of the other people who worked at the hospital. The time here had been well-spent. He wondered whether they would stay in contact much after they all finished their duty tours.

The rest of their time on base was eventful in many ways. Fred liked to fish and had grown up hunting birds and deer., These were plentiful in Montana, especially with his friend Frank's help. The whole family enjoyed trips to Yellowstone and to Glacier Park, and they managed to get up to Waterton Park, the Canadian part of Glacier Park. They considered traveling up to Canada's Banff and Jasper parks, but Wanda's pregnancy, and then miscarriage of their son, had put that on hold.

Other issues came up on the job. Fred was called to the site of a suicide by an airman. In another matter, he was asked to interview and evaluate the competence of an airman who was charged with murder. The incident involved an assault by one airman on another which led the second airman to arm himself. When he was accosted again and beaten badly, he shot his assailant. He claimed self-defense, but his problem was that he had gone back to the barracks to get his gun before their final encounter. He was found to be competent by Fred and was found guilty by the court martial. About six months into serving his sentence, he appealed, and on the retrial, he was acquitted. By that time most of the witnesses had been shipped out to other assignments and were unavailable to testify.

After spending two years in the Air Force, Fred was ready to move on. All he had to do was to decide what kind of practice he wanted to undertake. He and Wanda decided to go back to the university town where he had trained. It was familiar. There was a part-time job at the State Hospital, and he had an offer to partner with another psychiatrist in town. Wanda had contacts there, and Maria was eager to look up some old friends.

Chapter 42:
OUT IN THE CIVILIAN LIFE
November 1975

Fred and his family had been back in their Midwest university town for almost a year and a half. Fred had worked at the hospital for a while, but as his private practice picked up, he spent less time at the hospital, but did continue to do forensic work there. He was asked to consult on a case involving a young woman who had been stalking an older woman. Her defense attorney asked Fred to evaluate her for fitness to proceed to trial. There was a private investigator on the case whom Fred was asked to contact, because he had also been involved with the case for a while. The investigator was Karl Johnson. When Fred met with the investigator, it was none other than Clarence. They caught up over coffee, and Fred learned that Clarence had been hired by Ronald Torkensen, Maria's father, to work for him as an investigator for the newspaper. Clarence eventually went into business for himself and became reasonably successful as a private investigator, working primarily for attorneys. He was still in contact with Wilfred, who continued to work at the library but had begun to write some poetry of his own and published a couple of books.

In the case of the young woman about whom they were connecting, Clarence had some concerns and was glad that Fred was involved.

"She is off the beam, Dr. Q. She thinks the woman she was apparently stalking and trying to connect with is related to her in some weird way. I am glad that you are going to be looking at her. She even said that she was from some other planet, but when I tried to ask her what she meant, she clammed up. I found out a little about her background, Doc. She is in her early thirties and was raised in foster homes until she was eighteen. She was in some minor scrapes with the law, mostly misdemeanor stuff like petty theft, mostly of food items, trespassing after being told to leave an establishment, disorderly conduct, and indecent exposure. She apparently is fixated on this older woman, who volunteered at a food kitchen."

Fred arranged to have the woman brought to his office from the jail. She entered the office in a clean but simple dress, probably supplied by the jail staff. A female deputy lingered in the waiting room. Fred's desk faced the wall, about two feet from the door. When she entered with the deputy, Fred stood to introduce himself before excusing the deputy.

"Hello, I am Dr. Quimby. Can you tell me your name?"

"I am Susan Pile."

"Would you like to have a seat?" Fred pointed to a chair near the desk, situated so that he could both sit at the desk and write while facing her to his left. "Do you know why you have been sent to see me?"

"They think I'm crazy. Why else would they send me to see a shrink? I am not going to take any of your pills."

"I do not intend to give you any pills. I'm here to try to understand what got you into this mess, so I can help you out of it. So, what would lead anyone else to the idea that you are crazy?"

"They think that because I have run-ins with the cops all the time and I'm homeless, that I must be crazy, I guess."

"Do you know what you are charged with? Why you're in jail?"

"Yeah, I think that lady at the soup kitchen has something to do with it."

"Who is the lady at the soup kitchen? What's she got to do with all this?"

"I think she may be my mother, or at least my connection here."

"Tell me why you think that she may be your mother. Have you seen her before you met her at the soup kitchen?"

"She looks somehow familiar – she's got an aura about her. I feel connected to her in some way. She feels like we're from the same gene pool, either here or at home."

"At home? Where is home?"

"If I tell you that, you will think I'm nuts."

"Believe me, I have heard a lot of things that seem strange, but I don't just automatically think people are nuts. I try to find out why people do things, not just label them. You said she may be your mother or your connection here. Where is here, compared to there, and what kind of connection are you referring to?"

"I am not from this planet. I was put here to test me and to learn how to fit in for a special task that I am destined to do some time in the future. I will have a connection from my home planet, who will let me know the time and instruct me on what I am to do."

"So, is the woman at the soup kitchen your connection or your mother? Where does your mother come into this? My understanding, from what your attorney passed on to me, was that you were brought up in foster care until you were eighteen. Do you recall anything about your mother before being sent to foster care?"

"Apparently, I was given up for adoption, but it never worked out. I never met my mother until I saw her at the soup kitchen."

"So, this woman is either your mother or your connection to another planet. Do you know which? Could she be both? Or is she a kind person who spends her time in a soup kitchen helping others? Is she someone you would like to be connected with or be family with? Mistakes happen, and sometimes they work out well. Sounds like you have been alone for a good part of your life."

"See, you're trying to put a different spin on this."

"No, not really. I am trying to help you get to where you need to be, so that you don't end up in trouble and nobody gets hurt in the process. To do that, I have to understand what you are experiencing. You are already in trouble. I am just trying to help you find the best way out of the trouble you are in, and hopefully, to help you to not repeat it."

Susan was quiet. She looked wary and reluctant to say much more.

"Have you ever loved anyone, Susan?"

She remained quiet.

"I think you have. Maybe something happened to shatter your trust. Maybe something in the woman at the soup kitchen reminded you of that love and drew you in again. Was the woman kind?"

Susan's eyes watered and she turned her head.

Fred let that sink in for a moment and then said, "How do you know that I am not the connection who was sent to help you do what you need to do?"

Susan startled visibly and turned to look at him. Her demeanor reflected both amazement and disbelief.

"Is that possible?"

"You mentioned being tested. You don't want to give up an opportunity to learn what you need to learn. It is really up to you to find the answers you need and not throw away this opportunity."

Fred was careful not to say that he was her connection from another world, but left it enough of a question that he could keep her thinking about what life experiences may have led her to this bizarre thinking process. It appeared to be working.

She said, "Tell me more."

Fred said, "No, you tell me more."

Susan began to talk about her first foster mom and how kind she was, and the loss she experienced when the foster-mom got cancer, and Susan had to be placed elsewhere. She talked about some of the placements that were never quite right, and how she felt when she found out her original foster mother had died. She never had the opportunity to see her before it happened.

It was a tearful session, and arrangements were made for Fred to see her several more times before he had to submit a report. As she left, she looked at Fred and smiled just a little. "I think maybe I can trust you. We'll see."

Over the next ten days, Fred saw Susan three more times. He continued to softly lead her to understand that a lot of her obsession with the lady at the soup kitchen had to do with her genuine kindness, which Susan was missing in her life. She also gradually began to be able to see that if she wanted to have kindness come her way, it was up to her to be receptive to it. It was like the old saying, "Luck comes to those who have prepared themselves to receive it."

By the time he wrote the report to the court, there was still a question in Susan's mind whether she was supposed to have a "connection", and whether it might be this doctor. However, she was able to begin to grasp other aspects of her feelings, and it made sense to her to continue to explore this.

Fred's report recommended probation with the condition that she continue to work with a therapist.

The judge followed Fred's advice, put her on probation, and ordered her to make regular appointments at the local mental health clinic. He ordered her to have no contact with the lady at the soup kitchen. At the hearing, Susan cried and appealed to the judge to let her see Dr. Quimby instead of going to the clinic to start with a new person. She felt she could trust Dr. Quimby. The judge told her that the county could not manage the expense of a private psychiatrist, so, since she could not pay for it, and since the county had doctors and therapists on salary, seeing Dr. Quimby was not an option. Dr. Quimby spoke up and said, "Your honor, I would be willing to see her once a week for the next couple of months on a pro bono basis. I do think she has made some good progress in a short time and starting with another therapist might put a crimp in her healing."

"So be it. She's all yours, Dr. Quimby."

"Your honor, I would also like your permission to arrange supervised contact with Ms. Smith, the lady at the soup kitchen. It may help the process of healing."

The judge said, "A long as it is okay with Ms. Smith, you've got it, Dr. Quimby."

Chapter 43:
THE OTHER SIDE OF THE MOUNTAIN

Before Fred had started his training as a psychiatrist, he had interned in Denver. When he wanted a break from the city and the hospital, he would hop in the car and drive through the pass to the other side of the mountains. Things were less busy there. There were fewer people, and the fishing on that side of the Rockies was quieter and more productive. While Fred fished, he would sometimes imagine his late wife sitting on the bank with a sketch book and drawing quiet scenes. That was then, but Fred still referred to coming home from work and relaxing with Wanda and Maria as going to the other side of the mountain. He would still get an occasional call from a patient or a question from a colleague, but for Fred, home was peace. It may be busy, but it was family busy. It may be hectic, but it was his hectic.

Fred got home at about five-thirty, wondering what Wanda might have come up with for dinner. Fred often cooked on weekends, but Wanda usually figured out something during the week. Tonight, she decided to order a pizza. Fred was okay with that, but Maria was in one of her meatless moods, so Wanda tossed up a quick salad for her.

They sat down to have dinner together.

At the dinner table, Fred looked at them and said, "Remember Clarence, the guy who donated his marrow to Ron and then went to work with him for a while? Well, I have been working with him on a case for the court. I couldn't help but wonder how Ron is doing these days.

Wanda said, "I don't have a lot of contact with the family, but he seems to be over the hump with his leukemia. Work seems to be stressful. He's on a big case involving mob links."

Maria looked at her and asked, "What are mob links?"

Wanda looked at her and said, "That's when a bunch of people get together to do things that make money illegally."

Fred said, "Maybe he should get Clarence back on payroll to help out. But, on second thought, maybe that wouldn't be such a great idea." He thought to himself about the mafia fears and wondered whether Clarence still had his film tucked away in a safe deposit box.

The conversation continued on, covering a variety of topics; school, meat-eaters, careers, sports, friends, and homework. Maria commented on how a lot of her friends did not like math or science. She loved math and science.

Fred said, "Girls can be just as good or better at math and science as boys. During World War II, there were women in America who were doing important math and science for the government. In Britain, there were women who worked for their government and were experts at breaking the German codes. They saved a lot of lives."

Maria looked at him and said, "Well, my friends just don't think they are good at it, and so they don't try."

Wanda looked at her and said, "They probably don't think they are good enough at sports and other things, like art or music to try those either."

Maria looked at her and said, "That's about right."

Fred said, "You know, it is not how good you are at things, but how many things you try. The more things you experience, the better you are about knowing things. You can get to be super good at things, but it is important to learn other things as well, and to try out lots of things and not be afraid of them. The more things you try, the more about life you will learn, and the more you will enjoy life. As long, that is, that the things you try are not dumb things that we have told you not to do, right? OK, that was my sermon for the day."

Wanda chuckled and said, "We should get that one to the pastor for his sermon next Sunday, right, Maria."

Maria smiled, but said, "I think Fred is right. I like music, and I like sports, and I like math and science. I am not the best in the world, but I want to do them, and I want to learn about history and to read books. I want to do it all."

Wanda looked at her and said, "And no one in this family will ever stop you from doing that, but, …. you still have to do your chores."

After Maria had done her homework, had a bath and had gone to bed, Wanda looked at Fred with tears in her eyes and said, "I am so sorry, Fred, that we cannot have any more children. You are so good with them."

"Whoa, where is this coming from? I am perfectly happy with our family. We both had a rough time when you miscarried, but we still have each other and Maria."

"I was in touch today with an old friend who had lost her son in an accident, and I guess it brought up old feelings. Feelings that are old, but never go away."

"Some people come apart when they have a major loss, but I think our loss actually brought us closer together. It was a bad time, but the cement between us got firmer and more settled. I was actually thinking on my way from work today how relaxed and comfortable I feel when I know I am coming home."

"I sometimes cannot shake the feeling that you might be disappointed in me. I know that you don't blame me, but maybe I am disappointed in myself."

"Not a chance. You are my purpose. Without you, I would be a lonely guy, trying to figure out life. Please don't blame yourself for what nature has done. The miscarriage was no one's fault. We did all we knew to do to make the pregnancy work. Sometimes things happen, and we do not always know why. I don't blame you and couldn't be disappointed in you." Fred put his arms around Wanda and kissed her. "We have each other and Maria. We have friends. I am sure there will be others coming in and out of our lives that will become a part of us. My mother used to say that life is what goes on around us while we are planning other things. We have to pay attention to what is going on with us, not the other things."

Wanda looked at him through dewy eyes and said, "I am glad you married me. I am very lucky."

Fred said, "I am glad you made it easy for that to happen. I am the lucky one."

They cuddled contentedly on the couch for a while, then retired to the bedroom.

Chapter 44:
DOWN THE ROAD A BIT
September 1991

Fred was forty-nine and had been in his private practice now for seventeen years. By this time, Marie had finished college and had just graduated from law school. Wanda was still doing some nursing for a local clinic. Fred tried to mix his practice by doing some consulting at the university health service and at the local mental health clinic in addition to his private practice. He dealt with the usual medication management, but he continued to use hypnosis and other behavioral techniques to keep some variety in his work. A lot of his work consisted in working with families and couples. He also continued to get occasional calls from attorneys who wanted fitness evaluations for clients who might not be competent to stand trial for certain offenses.

All in all, Fred kept reasonably busy. On occasion, he would still run into Clarence, and he also had the opportunity on a couple of occasions to cross paths with John Maxwell. He had known John as Jonathon, as Jack, as Peter, and as Randolph. Jack had ended up as the dominant, though now more mature, personality as they had figured out the puzzle and gradually had become fused into one individual. At least they presented more fused now than when Fred had first met them at the hospital. John was now a policeman, so Fred would run into him from time to time in his court appointed work.

The first time Fred met up with John after moving back from the military, was an occasion when Fred was testifying on a case in court. After he was excused from the witness stand and started to leave the courtroom, a man in the gallery ran toward Fred with a knife in his hand, cursing all psychiatrists. A policeman quickly grabbed the man and disarmed him, then cuffed him and held him down until other officers joined him and took take he man away to jail. That cop happened to be John, who was formerly Jack some years before. As it turned out, one of his colleagues would evaluate the assailant and find him mentally ill and not fit to proceed with trial on the attempted assault. He was committed to a hospital for treatment. Fred also did not recognize the policeman, but John re-introduced himself to Fred, and they got together later to go over old times. The resident with whom Fred had left John at the state hospital, had enlisted the help of a senior staff member who specialized in hypnosis. He agreed with the plan that Fred had put forward, and together they managed to help integrate the different personalities to become much more functional together. Fred was grateful that things had turned out so well.

Fred had found over the years that hypnosis could be a quite useful tool to help people. He had a referral one day from another physician. The patient was a distinguished looking older retired man who introduced himself.

"Hello, Doctor. I was sent to see you by my doctor because I have terrible tinnitus. He wanted me to see you after I showed him my tinnitus pill."

Puzzled, Fred asked him what his tinnitus pill was.

The patient pulled a .38 caliber bullet out of his pocket.

They went on to talk about the man's work, which for many years, was operating heavy machinery. He had been very good at what he did, but it had taken a toll on his hearing over the years. Now he was unable to get the ringing sound out of his head and was at the end of his patience with it. Fred listened carefully. He saw that this man was respectful, attended to what Fred had to say, and seemed willing to do whatever he could to cooperate in his own treatment. Fred thought hypnosis might help.

Fred said, "I believe I can teach you some skills to alleviate the intensity of the sound that you are experiencing. As long as you can work with me in learning these skills, it should help."

Fred proceeded to talk to the patient in a calm low voice, gradually inducing a hypnotic state. He slowly got the man to relax, breathe calmly, and induced some simple post-hypnotic suggestions. During the hypnotic state, Fred suggested that the sounds the man was hearing would begin to take on a musical quality. Upon rousing him from the hypnotic state, the patient appeared much more relaxed and seemed confident enough in what had occurred, that he was willing to make further appointments to proceed with this treatment.

Over time, the man progressed to the point that Fred was able to teach him to use self-hypnosis. When he came in to see Fred, he would put himself into a trance in the waiting room, and he was able to use this calming effect in other situations as well. The ringing noise became much less intrusive and painful to him. He no longer wanted to leave the planet, and he was able to do some traveling and to take up some other hobbies. He and Fred agreed to keep in contact over time. On one occasion, he stopped by Fred's office to drop off a rock. He said,

"I arranged to take a float trip down the Grand Canyon. You are not supposed to take rocks or other things from the place, but I brought this one back for you, because now you will have to arrange to take a trip yourself and bring it back to the Grand Canyon for me. Enjoy the journey." About a month later, Fred learned that the man had died in his sleep. Fred was glad that his patient had the chance to enjoy that trip.

Fred used hypnosis from time to time when he judged it might be useful. A man he knew as an acquaintance came to him one day and told him that he wanted to quit smoking. Fred knew the man to be a rather controlled individual, so he wondered if this patient would be able to respond to someone inducing a state where he might feel he would be under someone else's control. Nonetheless, Fred suggested using hypnosis, and the man agreed to try it. Fred proceeded to speak in a calm quiet voice, getting the man to relax. He had him put his hands together and intermesh his fingers, suggesting that they would relax enough to feel as though they were like warm wax and had melted together. Fred began to give various suggestions about losing the urge to smoke. He watched the man attempt to pull his fingers apart and then give up as he focused more intently on Fred's suggestions. When Fred had finished, they talked about his experience.

"I was skeptical about this hypnosis thing, until I couldn't pull my hands apart."

Fred smiled and said, "This stuff can work, but it usually takes a few sessions to amplify the suggestions, especially in the early part of quitting smoking. We ought to schedule a few follow up sessions."

"I don't have my calendar with me, so I will have to call and schedule some time with your secretary."

The call never came, but Fred happened to run into him about a year later. He said, "I quit smoking, you know."

Fred smiled. "When did you stop?"

He said, "About a year ago."

It was clear that he had totally forgotten that he had come to see Fred and had a hypnotic experience.

Fred came to understand that hypnosis might work, but it did not always work toward the purpose he wanted. He had a patient who wanted him to hypnotize her to stop smoking. Fred found her to be very suggestible and a willing hypnotic subject. He left suggestions that every time she lit up, she would experience a terrible, foul taste. When she followed up with another visit, Fred asked her about her experience with smoking.

She said, "Whenever I lit up, I had the most awful taste in my mouth. It made me gag and want to throw up, but once I got past the first three or four puffs, I could manage the rest."

Fred concluded that she really did not want to stop smoking, and she probably would not be able to do so with this method.

Fred also saw families and children. He liked to work in different areas of interest. A man and his wife came to him about their five-year-old boy. They had recently had another child, and their first son was noted by his kindergarten teacher to be coloring all his pictures in black crayon. Thinking this might be related to having a new sibling, she told the parents about it. They wanted to bring him to a doctor.

Fred saw this youngster a couple days later. They sat down at a small table and Fred brought out crayons and paper and suggested they draw pictures. The child picked up the black crayon and started to draw. Fred said, "Wow you sure like the color black."

The child said, "Yeah, it's the same color as licorice, and that's my favorite candy."

It didn't take much more time to see that this child was not feeling displaced by his little brother. In fact, he was excited about him and looked forward to sharing his candy with him.

Fred saw teenagers as well. In one of his consulting jobs, he was appointed by the court to see a boy of sixteen, who was ordered to see a psychiatrist as part of his probation for assaulting a teacher. The boy was to see him weekly for at least ten sessions. The boy came to his office but sat sullenly and refused to interact with Fred, who tried for a while to engage him. Finally, he said, "You are stuck with having to come here every week for a while. If you don't want to talk, I have work to do at my desk. If you decide you want to talk, I will stop and listen. I'll leave it up to you."

They went on for several weeks this way with Fred working quietly at his desk. One day Fred ran into someone from the school who said, "I don't know what you are doing with that kid, but you have turned his behavior around a hundred and eighty degrees. He is a very cooperative and pleasant kid these days." Fred and the kid finished out the ten weeks. The kid never opened up to him. On the last day, the kid looked at Fred and said, "Thank you doctor, for not pressuring me. I think you know that things are better now." He reached out and shook Fred's hand. He then turned and walked out the door. Fred smiled.

At home things were going well. Fred and Wanda's nest was empty, but Marie visited when she could break away. She was married now, and the would-be grandparents hoped it would happen sometime soon.

Wanda had taken up oil painting with a passion and joined a hobby group that met weekly to try different styles and materials. It was a good social outlet and kept her immersed in many aspects of the art.

Fred liked to get away to fish when he could, but when he couldn't get away, his attempts at art involved his hobby of fly-tying.

Both of them liked to get out for walks and took cameras along to captivate, as well as they could, their experiences with nature. Wanda often used the photos as models for her paintings. Fred mainly just liked to look at them to reminisce about his walks with Wanda. Needless to say, coming home at night from the office was still for Fred, "going to the other side of the mountains."

Chapter 45:
CHANGE IN THE WIND
September 2004

Fred was now sixty-two. Wanda was a couple of years older at sixty-four. Life had been good to them. They were now grandparents to two children, Tommy age 9 and Chrissy age 7. They were able to see them at least a couple times a year and talked a lot by phone. As Fred and Wanda wandered into the 21st century, they also connected with Marie and her family by email and messages via computer. Fred wasn't rich, but he had accumulated enough money that they could be comfortable, and he was beginning to consider when he might retire, and what they would do if he did. Fred was at his office when he got a phone call that his secretary said he needed to take. It was a friend of Wanda, one of her fellow artists at her painting group.

"Fred, it's Jane. Wanda has been taken to the hospital. She was sitting at her easel mixing paints and collapsed on the floor. She had what looked like a seizure, and we immediately called 911. She's at University Hospital. I called you as they took her out."

The blood drained out of Fred's face. He said, "Oh my god, Jane. I'll get right over there." He hung up and said to his secretary, "Cancel the rest of my day. Wanda is in the hospital. I have to go. I will get back to you later."

Fred left immediately for the ER. By the time he arrived, Wanda had been sent to x-ray for tests. He asked to talk to the doctor, but he was busy with Wanda, so answers would have to wait on the test results. Meanwhile when she got back to her room, Fred would be able to wait by her bedside until they had some answers and a plan.

When the doctor appeared, Fred asked, "Was she conscious when she got here?"

The doc looked at him and said, "Sorry, Fred, she was not. It looked like she had had a neurovascular event. I have already alerted the neurosurgeon on call. As soon as we have some answers, I will let you know."

Fred tried to sit and wait, but he couldn't sit. He paced in the waiting area. Wanda's friend, Jane, soon showed up.

"What's happening, Fred? Do you know what her situation is? Are they working on her?"

"She's up in x-ray. Nothing yet. We have to wait till the tests come back. The doc will let me know as soon as he can."

Fred continued to pace.

The doctor showed up again after what seemed hours but was only about half an hour. He pulled Fred aside and said, "She has had an intracranial bleed. They sent her up immediately to the OR to relieve the pressure on her brain. Dr. Teller, our best neurosurgeon, is working on her. I would guess she will be in the ICU in about an hour. You will be able to go up there shortly after she gets there. I am sure Dr. Teller will give you all the details soon after that."

Fred went back to Jane and told her what the surgeon had told him. "It looks like she had a stroke with some bleeding. They took her to the OR. She will probably be there another hour or so. We'll know more after that."

Jane looked at Fred with tears in her eyes and said, "OK. I will wait here with you. I will need to call home and let them know that I will be here for a while."

The wait was agonizing. Fred paced, then sat, and paced again. Jane tried to hold back her tears so as not to make Fred's concerns worse. In about an hour and a half, Dr. Teller appeared in his scrubs.

"Dr. Quimby, the surgery went well. Your wife had a significant bleed into the left temporal area of her brain. We were able to stop the bleeding, but she has some significant swelling, so we will maintain her in a coma temporarily to allow things to settle down. You will be able to see her soon, but she will not be aware of your presence. It will be a few days before the swelling will resolve."

"Thank you, Dr. Teller. Can you tell me her prognosis? Will she have permanent effects?"

"I think you know as well as I, that we will not know the answer to those questions for at least a few days to a week or more. We will keep you tuned in to her progress as we go along. Meanwhile, after you check in on her in ICU, I would suggest that you make whatever arrangements that are needed for your practice and whatever contacts you need to make with friends and family. I know that you will want to be spending some time here with her and attending to personal issues. Now is the time for that. There is not a lot you can do here for now, other than pace and worry. We will take good care of her. She is not in any immediate danger."

"Thanks Doctor Teller. When can I see her?"

"They should get you up there sometime in the next half hour or so. You know the ICU. They will be hustling and bustling around her, so keep it short if you can. I will stay in touch with you about her progress over the next few days."

When he finally got to ICU, Fred saw the usual accouterments of the place. She had a heart monitor, was hooked to an EKG machine, an IV, oxygen hookup in her nose, and other instruments that were not familiar to Fred. Her eyes were closed. Her breathing was regular. He snuck in briefly between the nurses to hold her hand, but he quickly ducked back out of the way so he would not be hindering them in taking vital signs and other necessities. He asked if there were particular times that would be best to stop by to see her. He was told that he could stop by, but she would likely be in this condition for several days, so there would be no practical reason to stay for long periods of time. The doctor or head nurse could keep him informed of any changes in her condition.

Fred left the ICU and placed a call to Marie. She wanted to get on a plane to come right out, but Fred pointed out that she would just be sitting around waiting for her to become conscious. He convinced her to wait until the doctor said Wanda was ready. He assured her that he would call every day to let her know her progress and when she should come. Meanwhile, Jane, who had heard what Dr. Teller had told Fred, excused herself to go home to her family, and Fred agreed to keep her in the loop as well.

On the way out of the hospital, Fred heard a voice in the lobby.

"Got a dollar for a cup of coffee?"

Fred had not seen Clarence for several months. He was still busy with his private investigator business, but they had not had a common client in a long time.

"Sorry, Clarence, I am not in the mood for banter right now. Wanda is just out of surgery."

"Whoa, Doc, I am sorry. By the look on your face, it must be serious."

"Yes, she had emergency surgery and is in ICU."

"I have a friend in Admissions. I will keep tabs on her while she is here. If there is anything I can do to help, you know that you can count on me. Let me give you my card with my latest contact information on it. I will keep Wilfred in the loop as well, as long as that is OK with you."

"Fine, thanks, Clarence. I have to go now."

"Don't worry, Doc, I have enough cash for coffee. I will even buy you a cup, when you're ready, to help take the load off."

Wanda spent the next five days in ICU before she was stable enough to be moved to a surgical floor. She continued to be unresponsive, but Dr. Teller reassured Fred that she would likely regain consciousness. However he could not be sure yet, how much residual damage there would be. She would likely require a long course of physical therapy and perhaps speech therapy.

Fred came in daily to spend time with her. He would hold her hand and say a few words, but there was no response until one day she squeezed his hand slightly as he spoke to her. After that, he would talk to her a lot, reminding her about happy times together and encouraging her to get her strength back.

She had been on the ward about ten days when Fred came in earlier than usual and was surprised to see an older gentleman sitting by her bedside, reading to her. He thought at first that it might be a chaplain, but he saw that she was smiling. Then he noticed that it was Wilfred. Fred listened to the words of Emily Dickenson in Wilfred's deep and sonorous but gentle tone.

Hope is the thing with feathers
That perches in the soul,
And sings the tune without the words,
And never stops at all,

And sweetest in the gale is heard;
And sore must be the storm
That could abash the little bird
That kept so many warm.

I've heard it in the chillest land,
And on the strangest sea;
Yet, never, in extremity,
It asked a crumb of me.

Fred's eyes welled up. He had not seen a facial response from Wanda since her stroke. She was smiling. He was grateful to Wilfred for lighting up her soul again. He didn't say a word but just listened. He didn't want to break the spell.

Wilfred went on.

"And now my dear, to round out our visit, we'll have a little fun with an excerpt from Lewis Carroll's 'Jabberwocky' about the little boy who hunts the monster in his inimitable style."

He took his vorpal sword in hand;
    Long time the manxome foe he sought—
So rested he by the Tumtum tree
    And stood awhile in thought.

And, as in uffish thought he stood,
    The Jabberwock, with eyes of flame,
Came whiffling through the tulgey wood,
    And burbled as it came!

One, two! One, two! And through and through
    The vorpal blade went snicker-snack!

He left it dead, and with its head
   He went galumphing back.

Wilfred spoke the words with great flair and gusto as if he were on stage. Wanda's smile persisted. Then Wilfred spoke:

"Well, young lady, I must be off, but I shall return to read some more to you soon. We've had a lot of fun together today, haven't we?"

He turned to walk out and saw Fred.

"Oh, Dr. Quimby, I hope you don't mind my visiting my old nurse. Our friend, Clarence, told me she was here and would appreciate a little more company, so I have been reading a bit to her. She seems to enjoy it."

"Wilfred, I'm thrilled to see Wanda smiling. You have the magic touch. Please feel free to keep her company. When we have a chance, we ought to have a coffee and catch up. I am really grateful for your helping her. Great idea to read to her. I will have to bring some books myself."

Wilfred smiled and shook Fred's hand with both of his. He said, "Any help I can offer is my honor. You have done a lot for me." He turned and left the room.

In subsequent days, Fred found that reading short stories to Wanda seemed to help her respond. He thought he would leave the poetry mainly to Wilfred, who also came regularly to read to her. On one occasion, he approached her room and heard the plaintive tune of "Shenandoah" being played on a harmonica. It was a sad but moving song, and the melody suited the harmonica. He walked into Wanda's room just as Clarence was finishing playing. He could see the smile on her face, though her eyes remained closed. Clarence had tears in his eyes.

"She was always kind to me, Doc. I hope you don't mind my barging in to spend some time with her."

"Clarence, not at all. I am grateful to you for helping her spirit. Look, you made her smile."

"Doc, I will leave you with your wife, but I did schedule an appointment with you next week, if you will be working. There is something important I need to speak about with you."

"I will make it a point to keep that time available to you, Clarence. Meanwhile, thanks for the music."

Fred watched Clarence leave and pulled up a chair to Wanda's bed. He greeted her and she smiled, and then she opened her eyes for the first time since her hospitalization. She looked at him and tried to talk but struggled to make an utterance. Fred calmed her.

"Easy, easy, Wanda. It's okay, take your time. It's so good to see you. It will come. It might take a little time. I'll be here. Let it come naturally as your strength comes back. Maria was here, but she had to go back for a while. She will be coming again soon."

She smiled and squeezed his hand. He was grateful to have her back.

Chapter 46:
MAKING TIME FOR CLARENCE

Fred made it a point to keep the appointment with Clarence. It was the only business on his calendar, but he sensed some urgency in his voice, and Fred was grateful for his attention to Wanda. When he arrived, Clarence was in yet another of his many disguises. He wore jeans and a plaid shirt, and a fedora-like hat with long bleached hair attached. Fred felt the urge to compliment his new attire and its effect on his appearance, but instead, he said,

"OK, Clarence, another disguise. What's the occasion?"

"We're back to dealing with the mafia, Doc, but in an entirely different kind of way."

"And what kind of way is that, my friend?"

"Remember when we first talked about the mob? I was afraid they would try to kill me. I thought it was because I was seen as nosing around their business. I realize now that the information that I stumbled on in Mr. Fattorino's office was not a mob secret. It was Mr. Fattorino's secret from the mob. There was a lot of money missing that had to be stashed somewhere, and Mr. Fattorino knew exactly where it was and was not planning to tell anyone else about it."

"And how did you come to this conclusion?"

"Well, it seems that Mr. Fattorino met an untimely death without telling anyone else about his stash. The people who may have been involved in his untimely demise are now looking everywhere to get a clue as to where the missing cash could be. He apparently destroyed anything that could lead them to it before he departed this world. That leaves only me with that information. Moreover, I suspect the FBI might be very interested in getting that money back."

"How do you know all this?"

"I've been in this business a while now, Doc, and you know by now that I have my ways. Remember, I am not as dumb as I look."

"OK, Clarence, but why did you want to see me about this? In the past, you were always keeping me in the dark to protect me."

"Because after all these years, you would not be under suspicion by the mob, and I need a go-between to talk to my former boss, Mr. Torkensen, without putting him or his family in danger. I need his advice on who in the FBI that I can trust not to be connected to the mob. I still have those photos in a safe place. If I can get them safely to the Feds, about fifty million dollars could be returned, and I could finally get myself freed up from thinking about the mob all the time. Under the present circumstances, you would have a perfectly good reason to connect with him about Wanda and her daughter. Meanwhile, I may need to stay out of sight for a while, at least until the money is recovered. I will find a way to get in touch with you when the time is ripe. If you ever need to get in touch with me, put an ad in the Tribune that says, 'wanted - a used film camera' and use the old state hospital address. I will find you."

"So, I should get in touch with Torkensen and find out who is safe in the FBI, put an ad in the paper, and wait for you to find me?"

"That's right, Doc. You've got it down cold. I'll read the paper daily. Now, I have to skedaddle."

Fred watched him scoot out the door. "Oh boy, Clarence, another adventure. As if I didn't have enough on my hands right now."

He gathered up his things and followed Clarence out the door. His focus now had to be getting back to the hospital to see Wanda. He knew that she would be transferred to a rehab unit sometime soon. She was conscious and alert but had a long way to go with physical therapy, learning to walk and getting her speech back. Life would be different than they had expected, but they were lucky that she had survived, and he was grateful.

As he left the building, Fred had an uneasy feeling that he was being watched. He chalked it up to the relatively quiet street at this time of day and the mystique surrounding Clarence and his concerns about the mob. He couldn't help but wonder if the delusions were coming back for Clarence and considered starting him back up on medication at their next visit. Yet, there was a certain contagion of fear surrounding Clarence, and Fred wondered if he was just overreacting.

Chapter 47:
OLD DOGS LEARNING NEW TRICKS

Within a week, Wanda had been moved into neurology rehab and was getting workouts several times a day, learning to move parts that had been immobile, for the most part, since her cerebrovascular accident. When not working her muscles, she was being patiently, but persistently, encouraged to practice her word skills with a speech therapist. It would be a long haul, but she ground away like a trooper.

Fred tried to spend time with her when he knew she would have a respite from the therapists, which was mostly in the evenings. It allowed him to get some time in at the office, though he found it difficult to focus a lot of the time. He also managed to get to Mr. Torkensen to collect the information that Clarence wanted.

By now, Fred and 'Torky' were old friends, and he was eager to know how Wanda was doing and how Maria was taking it. Fred had no trouble filling him in on the challenges ahead and the relief that both he and Maria felt about her mother's recovery from a close call. Torky told Fred that it was good that Clarence was lying low until this thing was put into play by the FBI. He had been picking up rumblings from some of his informants that various individuals in the mob were indeed trying to get information on where the money ended up after Fattorino's untimely death. Apparently, they thought they knew where it was, but found out they were wrong after it was too late to extract the information from him. He told Fred to be careful and to keep a low profile with Clarence.

Fred left Torkensen's office. As he headed to his car, he noticed a man in a car across the street and had that same sense that someone was watching him. He tried to shrug it off, but after Torkensen's comments, he decided to be careful and to take an alternate route to the rehab center. He wanted to be able to more easily observe whether he was being followed. He made several turns and saw the same car making the same turns, though keeping its distance. Fred made a U turn and drove back the same way as though he had forgotten something. He passed the car and before it could turn around, Fred made a couple of quick turns down other streets. He didn't see the other car as he drove up to the rehab center.

Wanda was resting. She had just finished another punishing bout of physical therapy, but no matter how hard they worked her, she pushed her limits, knowing that it was the best way to get herself back to where she wanted to be. She had already come a long way with her ability to speak, though it was still halting. At least she could let him know what she wanted now, and they could carry on at least a semblance of a conversation.

Fred was told that the plan was to discharge Wanda to outpatient care in about a week, so both were excited. Fred knew, however, that it would mean changing his routine around, and that he would have to spend more time at home and away from the office. He had begun to start looking at retiring anyway, and perhaps just doing some occasional work for the courts, so this might be a good reason to ease into that kind of a routine. He stayed with Wanda for a couple of hours, but she was quite tired, so he left her to rest for the evening. He had been able to get the information from Torkensen that Clarence needed, so he needed to put together an ad for the paper and call it in the following morning.

On his way to the car, he noticed again, another car parked with the driver sitting inside. When he got to his car, he sat in it for a while. The other car waited, but when he started to pull out, the other car, after a short pause, also pulled out and began to go in the same direction. Fred decided not to drive home Instead he drove to the police station, parked and went in. Once inside, he spoke to the desk sergeant and said he wanted to donate to a program for young cadets aspiring to join the force someday. He wrote a check for twenty dollars, got a receipt, and left the station. The other car was nowhere in sight. He then drove the long way home, with a few minor detours, and felt that his ploy to spook the other car driver had worked, but the whole experience did raise his hackles a bit.

Chapter 48:
CONNECTING WITH CLARENCE

The ad went into the Tribune as planned – "wanted – a used film camera" with the address directed to the state hospital. When Fred got back to the rehab unit a couple of days later, one of the nurses handed him a letter that looked like an advertisement for a flower shop. The nurse said it was dropped off by a messenger on a bicycle. It was addressed to Dr. Fred Quimby, c/o Wanda Quimby, patient. Fred thanked the nurse and put the letter in his pocket. Later, when he had the opportunity, he opened it. Inside was a note from Clarence.

"Meet me at The Roadkill Grill on Fifth and Blair at 10 AM tomorrow, October 6. They have great coffee and food. We can talk safely there."

Fred wondered what kind of disguise Clarence would be wearing this time.

The next morning promptly at 10, Fred entered the Roadkill Grill. It was an old, converted railroad car with a long counter with stools and also a several booths opposite the counter. There were about half a dozen patrons in the place. Fred found a booth, hoping for some privacy, and sat down. A waitress came over to take his order. Fred just ordered coffee. The waitress returned with two coffees and two slices of coffee cake. She then sat down in the booth with Fred.

"Hi Doc. Looks like I did a good job with my makeup today."

Fred was truly surprised. He did not recognize Clarence in the waitress outfit. Fred gave him the information he needed that was passed along by Torkensen. They drank their coffee and ate the cake.

Clarence was just getting up when another patron walked over to the booth and sat down next to Fred. He said to the waitress, "Bring me a cup of that mojo and a piece of the cake too, please, and bring plenty of sugar. I like my coffee sweet."

Clarence returned shortly with the coffee and cake. He also brought a small bowl of sugar cubes. He then left the man sitting with Fred and returned back behind the counter.

The stranger looked at Fred and said, "I will wait here with you until your friend arrives."

Fred looked at him and said, "What friend are you talking about?"

"You know who I am talking about. The guy who knows where the money is." He put four lumps of sugar in his coffee, stirred it and began to sip. "Their coffee is as good as people say in this place."

Two policemen walked into the place and sat in one of the other booths. The stranger grew tense and told Fred to sit still and not say a word. The cops ordered coffee and coffee cake and carried on a conversation. The stranger continued to sip his coffee and signaled to the waitress to refill his cup. He added sugar cubes again. They sat for about fifteen minutes in silence while the police were on their break. The stranger began to sweat, his hands began to shake, he started to shiver, and he almost dropped his cup. The smallest sounds like spoons clinking startled him. He looked at Fred and said, "What the hell did you do to your face?"

Fred asked, "What do you mean?"

The stranger said, "Your face is moving around. It's melting. It's changing colors. And whatever they are cooking in the kitchen smells weird. It's making me feel sick. And what the hell is that dog doing in here?"

Fred looked at him and said, "What dog?"

The stranger pointed at the door. "That damn growling Doberman over there. He's coming this way." He pulled a gun out and shot twice in the direction he imagined the dog to be."

The police, who had just stood up to leave, quickly subdued and disarmed the man, called for backup, and arranged to get the stranger transported to a hospital. By this time, he was even more actively hallucinating. The police questioned Fred about him, but he was quite clear that he did not know the man, had never met him, and that the man was clearly psychotic. Once they found out Fred was a psychiatrist, they took his information so the doctors at the hospital could get more direct information from him.

After the police left, most of the clientele had left. Clarence came over to Fred and said, "It is a good thing that I happened to have some sugar cubes laced with acid and PCP. I knew the guy was up to no good. I saw the bulge under his shirt from the gun. He was looking for me. I need to get the information that I have to the FBI before something worse happens. I will get back to you when we are safe. Meanwhile, steer clear of me. I will be back in touch." Clarence managed to get himself disappeared rather quickly, and Fred took a powder as well. As it turned out,

Clarence had been right about his fears of the mafia all along.

Chapter 49: BREAKING NEWS

A week later, Fred opened the morning paper to find a startling headline:

$500 MILLION IN STOLEN MONEY RECOVERED BY FBI

The article did not mention how it was found, other than the fact that an individual, not to be named, was able to give the authorities some precise information that led to its discovery. The paper said no arrests were made at this time, but the investigation would be continuing. Evidence so far tended to be leaning in the direction of high placed officials with mob connections. The details were sparse, given the matter was still under investigation.

Fred had to admit to himself that he was surprised at the enormity of the whole enterprise. He had to chuckle to himself at how he had misjudged Clarence all along. Though he had not handled things well emotionally, it was clear that he had guessed right about the kind of danger he had feared. Fred wondered when Clarence might show up again.

About another week went by. Fred could see that Wanda was slowly making progress but knew it would be a long haul. He accepted that, but it was difficult to focus on issues at home and his practice at the same time. He preferred to be on "the other side of the mountains", but he still needed income to support their new caretaking expenses. He went to the mailbox and noted there was a letter with a foreign stamp. It was from Norway. It was addressed to "The honorable Dr. Fred Quimby" and sent to his home address. He went into the house and opened the letter. It was from Clarence. As he opened the folded letter, a piece of paper fell to the floor. Fred retrieved it and found it was a cashier's check for one million dollars. The letter read,

"Dear Dr. Q.,

Your support over all these years, even though you must have thought that I was nuttier than a fruitcake, has been both encouraging and sustaining. Both you and your wife, Wanda the nurse, as I liked to call her, have been kind and accepting of me. Now that she is recovering, thank God, from a serious life- threatening event, and clearly will need continued help, I have decided to share some of the reward money with you. I received said reward for my part in recovering the money that I am sure you read about in the news. The reward was substantial, so I can well afford to send this to you. I have also sent a surprise to Wilfred, so he can focus on his intellectual pursuits without having to putter around the library to get by. I, myself have decided to set up my own 'witness protection program' and will settle into my family's old stomping grounds for the near future to explore my roots. You will never know, however, when you might run into some stranger again looking for a handout.

Thanks again for all your help and understanding over many years, and until we meet again, have fun on the other side of the mountains.

Clarence"

Fred was flabbergasted. Over all these years that he had known Clarence, he had underestimated him. Yes, Clarence did suffer from paranoia, but, as it turned out, he had reason to be frightened, and, in the long run, he had played it well.

Chapter 50:
WINDING DOWN
June 2014

Wanda suffered another stroke in April of 2014. She did not come out of the coma after the second one, though she lingered for almost two months. It had given Fred some time to grieve while she was still alive. There were a lot of friends, and of course Marie and her family, at the funeral.

The ten years between the first and second stroke had been good ones. Fred had cut back his practice to one or two days a week, mostly doing consulting work. Clarence's beneficence had been most helpful in that regard. It allowed Wanda to get the therapy help she needed as well as getting help in the home.

At the funeral, people approached Fred and Marie's family to offer condolences. A gentleman with a goatee in a well-tailored suit approached Fred.

"Can I buy you a cup of coffee when things settle down?"

It was Clarence.

Fred replied, "Looks like you have done well for yourself, old friend. I would love to take you up on that."

Clarence asked, "Is it OK if I call you tomorrow, or would you want more time?"

"How about the day after tomorrow? Marie and her family will still be here, and I will want to be with them until they leave the next day."

"OK, I'll be in touch. I am really very sorry about Wanda. I would like to help you if I can. Meanwhile, take care of yourself and your family."

Clarence slipped out.

Two days later: It was about noon when Fred got a call on his cell phone. It was Clarence.

"Is this a good time to call, Doc? I wanted to make sure that I didn't wake you. Are you free to meet today? We could do lunch or dinner somewhere – your choice."

"I am free for the day, Clarence. My family has departed, so whatever works for you is fine with me."

They settled on a local pancake house.

"So, Clarence, how was Norway? It looks like it suited you well. I am really grateful that you came back for Wanda's funeral."

"Actually, the reason I came back was because I heard from Wilfred."

"I didn't see Wilfred at the funeral."

That's because he is also dying, Dr. Q."

Fred was taken aback. He had not expected to be thinking about another friend facing death.

"What is happening with Wilfred? What is he dying of?"

"He has pancreatic cancer."

"How much time does he have? Is it possible to see him?"

"He is conscious. He is getting medicine for pain, so he is often a bit sleepy, but if you want to see him, it should be soon. I saw him earlier this morning and mentioned you to him. He said that he would like to see you and talk to you."

Fred's eyes watered. He said, "To hell with breakfast, Clarence, let's go see him now."

They put the menus down and drove, with Clarence's direction, to the condo where Wilfred lived. He was in hospice and had some friends at his bedside. Fred approached gently as Clarence introduced him to Wilfred's friends. They made some room for Fred to get close, and Wilfred smiled at Fred.

"I'm glad to see you before I slip off into the sunset. Thank you, Doc, for all you did to help me find my new library and turn my life around."

"You told me once, professor, that you wished that you could have had me in some of your classes. The truth is, that I was a student of yours. I learned a great deal from you through our contacts."

"Then we learned from each other, Doc. You taught me how to let go of the unimportant things and find life again. I guess we were both students of each other and of life."

"I know we have not kept in close touch, Wilfred, but I will miss you."

"Don't you worry, Doc. I will be keeping an eye on you from another place."

"I certainly hope so. I will need all the oversight I can get, and I probably won't be that far behind you in the big picture."

"You just take care of yourself, Doc. There are still people out there just waiting to listen to your sage advice."

Fred could see that he was tiring.

"I wanted to say goodbye and thank you. I need to let you rest and continue with your friends. Have a peaceful journey. I will see you on the other side."

Wilfred smiled and nodded slightly. Fred got up and eased away from the bed. He and Clarence both wiped away tears on the way out.

EPILOGUE:
June 2021

    The old man once again entered the dog park with Sam, his dog. He watched the pooch sniff around until he relieved himself. He then picked up the small pile with a poop bag to deposit it in the garbage can left for that near the gate. They made their way to the park bench near the path that coursed the perimeter of the park. The weather was warm, but not too hot. The bench was in the shade. It was the time of day when people began to arrive with their pets. Sam was in the perfect spot. He could sniff the behinds of the various dogs as they went by and could lean against their human companions, hoping to get his rump and shoulders rubbed, or of mooching a treat. Young women seemed to be especially susceptible to Sam's entreaties.

    A young woman, hand in hand with a young man, looked particularly familiar to Fred as she approached on the path. He realized it was the student he had encountered three months previously. It was clear that she was entranced with her companion. Fred wondered if this was the man she railed against when they spoke, or if it was another romantic interest. He was curious, but he was not about to engage her unless she approached him. As the couple walked by, Sam made the introduction. He approached the couple with his doggy grin and waving tail. The young lady leaned down to pet him and said, "Sam! You're here." She looked up toward the bench and saw the old man and smiled. "And your buddy is here." She looked at her companion and said, "This is the man I told you about. It's funny. I know his dog's name, but I never asked him his name. I almost didn't recognize him with the hat and sunglasses. All I know is that he worked at the university as a psychiatrist, and I unloaded on him about personal issues. He listened patiently and gave me good advice. I slept well that night for the first time in a long while. I wondered whether he hypnotized me or something, because I have been more relaxed since we talked. Nice to see you again, Doctor -------?"

"Just call me Fred, and no, I did not hypnotize you. I just suggested that you make the best choices you could with the information at hand and live with those choices and learn from your mistakes. Sounds like you did just that. No magic involved."

Fred thought to himself – no hypnosis, just suggestion, the basis of hypnosis.

"But you steered me in the right direction."

"And you accepted yourself and trusted your decisions."

"I want you to meet my new friend, Jimmy. We've been dating for about two months, now. He's in pre-med."

"Nice to meet you, Jimmy. Looks like you are lucky enough to be dating a woman who can look after herself."

Jimmy looked at the old man and said, "I am grateful that you helped Miriam to find herself. I am lucky to have found her. She is wonderful to be with."

"Well, we had a fortuitous encounter. I am glad that we had the chance to talk. I am glad it was helpful. It seems we were in the right place at the right time."

She looked at Fred and said, "Call it what you want, luck, angels, spirits, whatever; I am glad we had that opportunity. Your words were helpful, and I am thankful. That other issue we talked about is now well in the past."

She squeezed Jimmy's hand and leaned into him and said, "We'd better be on our way and leave him alone. I about talked the man's ears off the last time."

Fred surmised that she did not want to continue the discussion that could lead into her "other issue".

The couple proceeded along the perimeter path. She looked back over her shoulder at Fred, smiled, and gave a short wave as she mouthed the words, "Thank you" as they continued to walk on.

Fred knew it was also time for him to move on. He looked at Sam and said, "Let's go buddy, it's time for us to head home." He stood up and started his walk to the gate. Sam obediently followed.

Fred was pleased to know that the seeds that he had planted had been helpful. He knew that the timing had been right, and that she had also been ready to hear what he had to say. Psychiatry, like farming, depends on when to do the planting, but the soil also needs to be ready.

Fred looked at Sam as they got to the gate.

"Well, Sam, what now? Back to an empty house? What's next? More TV? Read another novel? Plan a fishing trip? Get the camera out and go take photos? Play poker with friends? Take up the banjo?"

Quimby's quandary was – where to take his life from here. He was an old man. His wife was gone. His remaining family was not around. It was just Fred and Sam. Sure, he had friends, but they had their lives, and poker once or twice a month didn't do it all.

"Well, Sam, I guess maybe it's time to write my own book! That'll keep me busy for a while."

Acknowledgements to those who helped guide me through the writing of Quimby:

Thanks to Pete Swan who pushed his way through over three hundred pages of recommended grammar and readability notations, with lots of good advice.

Thanks to Duncan and Denise Rutter and to Ernie and Kathy Deacon for reading the first draft and encouraging me.

Thanks to David Diethelm for his patience with me in getting things together for publication and encouraging me.

And --- thank you to my wife, Judy, who is now gone, but who patiently went through many of the experiences with me that I have somewhat fictionalized in this book.

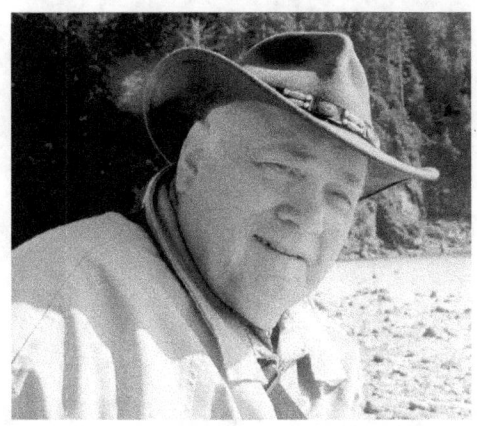

Jerome Vergamini M.D. is a retired psychiatrist who was raised in northern Wisconsin, went to small colleges in Minnesota, and got his medical degree at the University of Wisconsin-Madison in 1965. He finished a one-year rotating internship at St. Joseph Hospital in Denver and returned to University Hospitals in Madison for a three-year residency in psychiatry.

In 1969, the Viet Nam war was continuing. Dr. Vergamini was called into the US Air Force and was assigned to a missile base in Montana. Two years later, when his service ended, he returned to northern Wisconsin to serve as medical director and administrator to a small mental health clinic. After two years an opportunity came up to return for more training as a child psychiatrist. After completing two more years of training, he accepted an opportunity to practice in Eugene, Oregon, where he lives and worked until his retirement in 2020, as the Coronavirus pandemic exploded.

His practice over the years has included consultation to the courts and to numerous residential and outpatient treatment programs for children and adolescents. He has served on the board of the Oregon Psychiatric Association and served as president of that organization for one year. He was chief of psychiatry at Sacred Heart Hospital for a one-year term.

Dr. Vergamini had been married to the same woman for 56 years, until her death in 2021. They have three grown children and two grandchildren. This is his second book. The first, *A Fieldguide to the American Teenager, A Survival Guide for Parents,* was published in 2016, with co-author Ray Miskimins Ph.D.

www.ingramcontent.com/pod-product-compliance
Lightning Source LLC
Chambersburg PA
CBHW081743100526
44592CB00015B/2285